Treatment of
Recurrent Depression

D1227586

Review of Psychiatry Series
John M. Oldham, M.D.
Michelle B. Riba, M.D., M.S.
Series Editors

Treatment of Recurrent Depression

EDITED BY

John F. Greden, M.D.

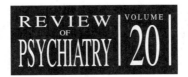

No. 5

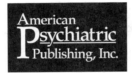

Washington, DC
London, England

Copyright © 2001 American Psychiatric Publishing, Inc.
04   03   02   01   4   3   2   1

ALL RIGHTS RESERVED
Manufactured in the United States of America on acid-free paper
First Edition

American Psychiatric Publishing, Inc.
1400 K Street, NW
Washington, DC 20005
www.appi.org

The correct citation for this book is

> Greden JF (editor): *Treatment of Recurrent Depression* (Review of Psychiatry Series, Volume 20, Number 5; Oldham JM and Riba MB, series editors). Washington, DC, American Psychiatric Publishing, 2001

Library of Congress Cataloging-in-Publication Data
Treatment of recurrent depression / edited by John F. Greden.
     p. ; cm. — (Review of psychiatry ; v. 20, n. 5)
    Includes bibliographical references and index.
    ISBN 1-58562-025-4 (alk. paper)
    1. Depression, Mental. 2. Depression, Mental—Treatment. I. Greden, John F., 1942–   II. Review of psychiatry series v. 20, 5.
    [DNLM: 1. Depressive Disorder—therapy. 2. Depressive Disorder—prevention & control. 3. Recurrence—prevention and control. WM 171 T7844 2001]
RC537 .T742 2001
616.85'2706—dc21

                                       00-069520

British Library Cataloguing in Publication Data
A CIP record is available from the British Library.

Cover illustration: Copyright© 2001 Amy DeVoogd/Artville.

*Dedicated to those caring, magnanimous
individuals who support the research
necessary to conquer depression*

Contents

Chapter 3

Chronic and Recurrent Depression:
Pharmacotherapy and Psychotherapy Combinations **59**
Robert Boland, M.D.
Martin B. Keller, M.D.

Chapter 4

Prevention of Recurrences in Patients With Bipolar
Disorder: The Best of the Old and the New **81**
Charles L. Bowden, M.D.
Cheryl L. Gonzales, M.D.

Contributors

Berry Anderson, R.N.
Research Nurse, Brain Stimulation Laboratory and Center for Advanced Imaging Research, Departments of Psychiatry, Radiology, Neurology, and Neurosurgery, Medical University of South Carolina, Charleston, South Carolina

Robert Boland, M.D.
Assistant Professor, Department of Psychiatry and Human Behavior, Brown University, Providence, Rhode Island

Charles L. Bowden, M.D.
Professor and Chairman, Department of Psychiatry, University of Texas Health Science Center at San Antonio, San Antonio, Texas

Jeong-Ho Chae, M.D.
Visiting Scientist, Brain Stimulation Laboratory and Center for Advanced Imaging Research, Departments of Psychiatry, Radiology, Neurology, and Neurosurgery, Medical University of South Carolina, Charleston, South Carolina; Assistant Professor, Catholic University of Korea, Seoul, Korea

Heather A. Flynn, Ph.D.
Assistant Research Scientist, Department of Psychiatry, University of Michigan, Ann Arbor, Michigan

Mark S. George, M.D.
Distinguished Professor of Psychiatry, Radiology and Neurology, Brain Stimulation Laboratory and Center for Advanced Imaging Research, Departments of Psychiatry, Radiology, Neurology, and Neurosurgery, Medical University of South Carolina, Charleston, South Carolina

Neera Ghaziuddin, M.D.
Assistant Professor, Child and Adolescent Psychiatry, Department of Psychiatry, University of Michigan, Ann Arbor, Michigan

Cheryl L. Gonzales, M.D.
Assistant Professor, Department of Psychiatry, University of Texas Health Science Center at San Antonio, San Antonio, Texas

John F. Greden, M.D.
Rachel Upjohn Professor of Psychiatry and Clinical Neurosciences; Chair, Department of Psychiatry; Senior Research Scientist, Mental Health Research Institute; and Director, The University of Michigan Depression Center, The University of Michigan, Ann Arbor, Michigan

Martin B. Keller, M.D.
Professor and Chair, Department of Psychiatry and Human Behavior, Brown University, Providence, Rhode Island

Xing-Bao Li, M.D.
Visiting Scientist, Brain Stimulation Laboratory and Center for Advanced Imaging Research, Departments of Psychiatry, Radiology, Neurology, and Neurosurgery, Medical University of South Carolina, Charleston, South Carolina; Associate Professor, Shandong University, Jinan, Shandong, China

Sheila M. Marcus, M.D.
Director, Adult Ambulatory Division, Department of Psychiatry, University of Michigan, Ann Arbor, Michigan

Sharon Mudd, M.S., R.N., C.S., N.P.
Nurse Practitioner, Department of Psychiatry, University of Michigan, Ann Arbor, Michigan

Ziad Nahas, M.D.
Assistant Professor, Brain Stimulation Laboratory and Center for Advanced Imaging Research, Departments of Psychiatry, Radiology, Neurology, and Neurosurgery, Medical University of South Carolina, Charleston, South Carolina

Arif Najib, B.S.
Exchange Student, Brain Stimulation Laboratory and Center for Advanced Imaging Research, Departments of Psychiatry, Radiology, Neurology, and Neurosurgery, Medical University of South Carolina, Charleston, South Carolina

John M. Oldham, M.D.
Dollard Professor and Acting Chairman, Department of Psychiatry, Columbia University College of Physicians and Surgeons, New York, New York

Nicholas Oliver, B.S.
Research Associate, Brain Stimulation Laboratory and Center for Advanced Imaging Research, Departments of Psychiatry, Radiology, Neurology, and Neurosurgery, Medical University of South Carolina, Charleston, South Carolina

Michelle B. Riba, M.D., M.S.
Associate Chair for Education and Academic Affairs, Department of Psychiatry, University of Michigan Medical School, Ann Arbor, Michigan

Elizabeth A. Young, M.D.
Professor and Research Scientist, Department of Psychiatry, University of Michigan, Ann Arbor, Michigan

Introduction to the Review of Psychiatry Series

John M. Oldham, M.D., and
Michelle B. Riba, M.D., M.S., Series Editors

2001 REVIEW OF PSYCHIATRY SERIES TITLES

- *PTSD in Children and Adolescents*
  EDITED BY SPENCER ETH, M.D.
- *Integrated Treatment of Psychiatric Disorders*
  EDITED BY JERALD KAY, M.D.
- *Somatoform and Factitious Disorders*
  EDITED BY KATHARINE A. PHILLIPS, M.D.
- *Treatment of Recurrent Depression*
  EDITED BY JOHN F. GREDEN, M.D.
- *Advances in Brain Imaging*
  EDITED BY JOHN M. MORIHISA, M.D.

In today's rapidly changing world, the dissemination of information is one of its rapidly changing elements. Information virtually assaults us, and proclaimed experts abound. Witness, for example, the 2000 presidential election in the United States, during which instant opinions were plentiful about the previously obscure science of voting machines, the electoral college, and the meaning of the words of the highest court in the land. For medicine the situation is the same: the World Wide Web virtually bulges with health advice, treatment recommendations, and strident warnings about the dangers of this approach or that. Authoritative and reliable guides to help the consumer differentiate between sound advice and unsubstantiated opinion are hard to come by, and our patients and their families may be misled by bad information without even knowing it.

At no time has it been more important, then, for psychiatrists and other clinicians to be well informed, armed with the very latest findings, and well versed in evidence-based medicine. We have designed Volume 20 of the Review of Psychiatry Series with these trends in mind—to be, if you will, a how-to manual: how to accurately identify illnesses, how to understand where they come from and what is going wrong in specific conditions, how to measure the extent of the problem, and how to design the best treatment, especially for the particularly difficult-to-treat disorders.

The central importance of stress as a pathogen in major mental illness throughout the life cycle is increasingly clear. One form of stress is *trauma*. Extreme trauma can lead to illness at any age, but its potential to set the stage badly for life when severe trauma occurs during early childhood is increasingly recognized. In *PTSD in Children and Adolescents,* Spencer Eth and colleagues review the evidence from animal and human studies of the aberrations, both psychological and biological, that can persist throughout adulthood as a result of trauma experienced during childhood. Newer technologies have led to new knowledge of the profound nature of some of these changes, from persistently altered stress hormones to gene expression and altered protein formation. In turn, hypersensitivities result from this early stress-induced biological programming, so that cognitive and emotional symptom patterns emerge rapidly in reaction to specific environmental stimuli.

Nowhere in the field of medicine is technology advancing more rapidly than in brain imaging, generating a level of excitement that surely surpasses the historical moment when the discovery of the X ray first allowed us to noninvasively see into the living human body. The new imaging methods, fortunately, do not involve the risk of radiation exposure, and the capacity of the newest imaging machines to reveal brain structure and function in great detail is remarkable. Yet in many ways these techniques still elude clinical application, since they are expensive and increasingly complex to administer and interpret. John Morihisa has gathered a group of our best experts to discuss the latest developments in *Advances in Brain Imaging,* and the shift toward greater clinical utility is clear in their descriptions of these methods. Perhaps most intriguing is the promise that through these methods we can identify, before the onset of symptoms, those most at risk of developing psychiatric disorders, as discussed by Daniel Pine regarding childhood disorders and by Harold Sackeim regarding late-life depression.

Certain conditions, such as the somatoform and factitious disorders, can baffle even our most experienced clinicians. As Katharine Phillips points out in her foreword to *Somatoform and Factitious Disorders*, these disorders frequently go unrecognized or are misdiagnosed, and patients with these conditions may be seen more often in the offices of nonpsychiatric physicians than in those of psychiatrists. Although these conditions have been reported throughout the recorded history of medicine, patients with these disorders either are fully convinced that their problems are "physical" instead of "mental" or choose to present their problems that way. In this book, experienced clinicians provide guidelines to help identify the presence of the somatoform and factitious disorders, as well as recommendations about their treatment.

Treatment of all psychiatric disorders is always evolving, based on new findings and clinical experience; at times, the field has become polarized, with advocates of one approach vying with advocates of another (e.g., psychotherapy versus pharmacotherapy). Patients, however, have the right to receive the best treatment available, and most of the time the best treatment includes psychotherapy *and* pharmacotherapy, as detailed in *Integrated Treatment of Psychiatric Disorders*. Jerald Kay and colleagues propose the term *integrated treatment* for this approach, a recommended fundamental of treatment planning. Psychotherapy alone, of course, may be the best treatment for some patients, just as pharmacotherapy may be the mainstay of treatment for others, but in all cases there should be thoughtful consideration of a combination of these approaches.

Finally, despite tremendous progress in the treatment of most psychiatric disorders, there are some conditions that are stubbornly persistent in spite of the best efforts of our experts. John Greden takes up one such area in *Treatment of Recurrent Depres-*

sion, referring to recurrent depression as one of the most disabling disorders of all, so that, in his opinion, "a call to arms" is needed. Experienced clinicians and researchers review optimal treatment approaches for this clinical population. As well, new strategies, such as vagus nerve stimulation and minimally invasive brain stimulation, are reviewed, indicating the need to go beyond our currently available treatments for these seriously ill patients.

All in all, we believe that Volume 20 admirably succeeds in advising us how to do the best job that can be done at this point to diagnose, understand, measure, and treat some of the most challenging conditions that prompt patients to seek psychiatric help.

Chapter 1

Recurrent Depression

Its Overwhelming Burden

John F. Greden, M.D.

Depression, when recurrent, is usually overwhelmingly burdensome. The World Health Organization (WHO) ranked all major medical disorders in the world by disability adjusted life years (DALY), a new, standardized measure of burden. Major depressive disorder (MDD) was ranked the fourth most disabling, and bipolar disorder was ranked sixth (Murray and Lopez 1996). WHO projected that by 2010, MDD will be ranked second unless meaningful improvements occur in prevention, diagnosis, and treatment. The disability MDD induces in women is even greater, ranking first for major age groups. When other disabilities, global measures of burden, and bipolar disorder are considered, MDD is arguably one of the most disabling disorders in the world.

The burden of depression is buttressed by powerful epidemiological data, such as the number of people who have the disorder, mortality rates from suicide, personal and familial consequences, and financial costs. More than 340 million people worldwide and 18 million people in the United States alone are estimated to have depression at any one time (Murray and Lopez 1996). Teen suicides, long a concern (Pfeffer 1992), in the United States have increased fourfold in the past several decades, ranging from a low of 2.3 per 100,000 in 1956 to 9.5 per 100,000 in 1997 (Koch 2000). Depressed patients' health care expenditures have skyrocketed and are commonly estimated to be several-fold higher than those for nondepressed patients, *not* counting mental health costs

(Kamlet et al. 1993; Mintz et al. 1992). Corporations, other businesses, and insurance providers are losing vast amounts of money as a result of impaired work performance, absenteeism, medical visits, hospitalizations, and other expenses associated with unresolved depression (Mintz et al. 1992). In fact, U.S. businesses have found that high health care costs for employees and retirees are predominantly attributable to care required by individuals with five "high-utilizing" diseases, often coexisting: cardiovascular problems, depression, diabetes, substance abuse, and airway illnesses such as asthma and emphysema. This recognition has led to development of specific, integrated disease management programs for individuals with these conditions. Such programs illustrate the growing recognition of the burden of depression on society.

Although there are many contributors to the high morbidity of MDD, recurrences of MDD are perhaps the most important. If we are to reduce the personal and societal consequences and costs of MDD, we must tackle the problem of recurrences. That is the focus of this book.

Emphasis will be placed on five topics:

1. Women, because they have the highest prevalence and experience the heaviest burden (see Chapter 2)
2. Treatment strategies for chronic and recurrent depression, specifically whether pharmacotherapy and psychotherapy in combination are superior to either treatment alone (see Chapter 3)
3. Prevention of recurrences of bipolar disorder, particularly in light of the fact that a number of new anticonvulsant mood stabilizers have been introduced and that integrative treatment approaches appear to be beneficial (see Chapter 4)
4. Potential applications of new somatic treatment strategies, particularly in light of the fact that data suggest vagus nerve stimulation (VNS) and repetitive transcranial magnetic stimulation (rTMS) may join our treatment armamentarium (see Chapter 5)
5. An update of recommendations to help us make progress in preventing recurrences of depression, emphasizing that noth-

ing short of paradigm shifts will suffice, nothing short of a "call to arms" (see Chapter 6)

Figure 1–1 presents contributors to the overwhelming burden of MDD. These will be reviewed briefly, followed by a discussion of strategies to overcome or prevent them.

Widespread Prevalence

The lifetime prevalence of depression was assessed in a large national sample by Kessler et al. (1994). The authors determined that 12.7% of males had a lifetime risk for MDD, whereas for women this figure rose to 21.3%. When mania episodes and chronic minor depression were incorporated, the lifetime risks for men and women rose to 19.1% and 31.0%, respectively. With a disorder so prevalent and disabling, clinicians in primary care settings must become more attuned to its possible presence.

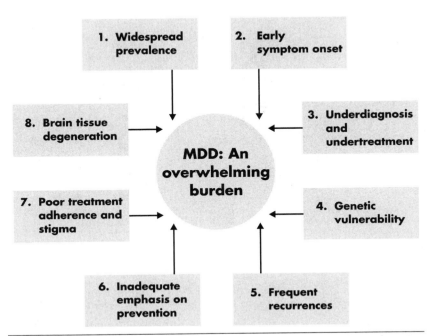

Figure 1–1. Contributors to the overwhelming burden of major depressive disorder (MDD).

Early Symptom Onset

Symptom onset for those who develop MDD or bipolar disorder commonly occurs in late adolescence. Peak ages at onset appear to be 15–19 years (Pine et al. 1998; Roy-Byrne et al. 1985). Rarely is a diagnosis of depression made because of the presence of prodromal symptoms. Rather, these patients' disorders are diagnosed as "adjustment disorders of adolescence" or attention-deficit/hyperactivity disorder (ADHD), or the clinician focuses on coexisting substance abuse. Meanwhile, the primary underlying depression goes undiagnosed and untreated. This failure to detect and intervene early is arguably the beginning of the pattern of lifelong morbidity of MDD.

The high prevalence of MDD in women is associated with early age at onset. The National Comorbidity Survey (NCS; Kessler et al. 1994) revealed that women are approximately 1.7 times more likely to report a lifetime history of MDD than men, and age-at-onset analysis revealed that this difference begins in early adolescence. Kessler et al. (1993) concluded that the 12-month prevalence of depression among women largely resulted from their higher risk of early onset.

When onset is early and undetected, the patient is at greater risk for increasing problems in subsequent years. Pine et al. (1998) noted that patients with subclinical depressive symptoms during adolescence had a two- to three-times greater risk for adult MDD. For adolescents whose symptoms are more severe—and as many as 1 in 33 children and 1 in 8 adolescents have symptoms that actually meet the criteria for diagnosis of MDD—early-onset untreated MDD is also associated with longer-lasting index episodes, higher rates of recurrence, higher rates of comorbid personality disorders, lifetime substance use disorders, greater numbers of hospitalizations, and a greater family history of mood disorders (Klein et al. 1999).

Early subclinical depression or MDD appears to affect the sexes differently. Berndt et al. (2000) reported that lower educational attainment and lower annual earnings were associated with 12%–18% of women with early onset, but that these two factors were not associated with men who had early onset. These and other findings justify that special attention be given to depression among women. It is reasonable to infer that among both sexes, untreated early subclinical depression or MDD, the growing co-morbidity of substance abuse, and the burgeoning availability of guns (Pfeffer 1986) are key interactive factors in the distressing increase in teen suicide rates over the past several decades. Failure to detect and treat subclinical depression or full-fledged MDD during childhood and adolescence is not only burdensome to the patient but sometimes lethal.

Many or most of the negative consequences of MDD could be averted or minimized if MDD is detected and treated earlier and the patient's wellness is maintained. For this to occur, clinicians must ensure that MDD is treated early, particularly among children and adolescents. Pine et al. (1998) asserted that when children and adolescents have symptoms of depression, their families, friends, teachers, and clinicians need to consider the possibility that they have a mood disorder, not just "moodiness." For success in stopping progression, we first must have success in improving detection. Then we can continue our efforts to understand how children and adolescents with MDD differ from adults with MDD in their underlying neurobiology and in their response to treatment (Ghaziuddin et al. 2000).

Underdiagnosis and Undertreatment

Failure to detect early depression is complicated by severe underdiagnosis and undertreatment. In 1996 the National Depressive and Manic-Depressive Association (National DMDA) held a conference to review the adequacy of diagnosis and treatment of depression (Hirschfeld et al. 1997). Participants concluded that there was overwhelming evidence that individuals with depression were seriously undertreated. Reasons included an array of patient, health care provider, and health care system factors.

Some patients who are undertreated for depression actually get no treatment. Others are treated with medications or psychotherapies that are not demonstrated to effectively treat MDD. Perhaps the most perplexing offender is preferential use of benzodiazepines. Another form of inadequate treatment is one that leads to incomplete recovery. Whatever the reasons, Judd et al. (2000) revealed that patients with residual subthreshold depressive symptoms during recovery had significantly more severe and chronic future courses, faster relapses to major and minor depressive episodes, more recurrences, shorter intervals of wellness, and fewer symptom-free weeks. This can mean the beginning of a patient's lifelong burden and disability resulting from undertreated, recurrent MDD. The dramatic differences between patients with complete versus incomplete remission are illustrated in Figure 1–2. Clinicians must strive not only to recognize and treat MDD early but also to treat it adequately. Severe underdiagnosis and undertreatment encourage high morbidity and even mortality.

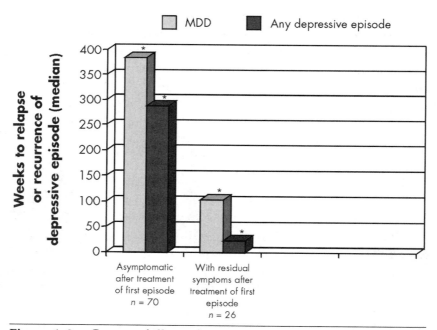

Figure 1–2. Course of illness for patients with and without residual symptoms following treatment for first episode of major depressive disorder (MDD).

*P<0.0001.

Source. Data from Judd LL, Paulus M, Schettler P, et al.: "Does Incomplete Recovery From First Lifetime Major Depressive Episode Herald a Chronic Course of Illness?" *American Journal of Psychiatry* 157:1501–1504, 2000.

Genetic Vulnerability

Genetic vulnerability appears to play a role in recurrences of depression. Kendler et al. (1993b, 1999) reported that stressful life events are correlated with genetic vulnerabilities and that when stressors occur, the risk of another episode of MDD increases significantly. Several practical questions emerge: Can we avoid stressors? What factors underlie stress-genetic interactions, and do they have treatment implications? Are there ways to identify individuals with genetic vulnerabilities and intervene to prevent MDD?

Can We Avoid Stressors?

Unfortunately, it is not possible to avoid stressors. We need to do what we can, but realistically, the clinician needs to shift attention from lamenting unavoidable stressors and recurrences to providing wellness maintenance for those with underlying genetic vulnerabilities and previous episodes of depression. Only then is it possible to prevent recurrences when stressors do emerge.

What Factors Underlie Stress-Genetic Interactions, and Do They Have Treatment Implications?

Lopez et al. (1998) and Zimmer (2000) have determined that there are significant differences between male and female rats in the way they respond to stress and that both serotonin (5-HT) and estrogen help regulate stress response. The researchers found post-stress steroid hormone levels (corticosterone) to be much higher in female rats than males and observed that 5-HT receptors (5-HT_{1A} and 5-HT_{2A}) are resistant to chronic stress-induced alterations in female animals. Of relevance for clinicians, fluoxetine, a selective serotonin reuptake inhibitor (SSRI) antidepressant, was found to be more efficient than the tricyclic antidepressant desipramine in preventing stress-induced alterations of the hypothalamic-pituitary-adrenal (HPA) axis in female animals. SSRI administration helped prevent alterations of the estrous cycle induced by chronic stress. The complexity of this interface is revealed by the fact that estrogen administration during nonstress conditions elevates resting levels of corticosterone, whereas estrogen given during chronic stress prevents increases in stress hormones.

More studies need to be conducted, but the data above suggest potential for clinical practice, implying that 1) estrogen may have "antidepressant" actions in an animal model of chronic stress; 2) antidepressant effects may occur partially through inhibition of the HPA axis; 3) females and males may respond differently to different antidepressant classes, with females more favorably affected by SSRIs than males; and 4) studying estrogen/stress/ serotonergic interactions may have implications for new treatment strategies. Pursuit of these topics is promising.

Are There Ways to Identify Individuals With Genetic Vulnerabilities and Intervene to Prevent Recurrences of MDD?

It is now reasonable to expect that clinicians of the future "may treat diseases in much the same way that software engineers fix a faulty computer program: by isolating flaws in the code. . . . If the effort is successful, healthcare will shift from a paradigm of detect and treat, typically with toxic drugs that sometimes do no more than mask symptoms to predict and prevent, with therapies of exquisite specificity aimed at the causes of disease" (Fisher 1999). While we are working to make that happen, we must still employ clinical strategies to minimize the impact of MDD: 1) clinically detecting individuals who have a positive family history or have had previous episodes of MDD; 2) working with vulnerable individuals to help them avoid stressors as much as possible; 3) teaching individuals how to cope better with severe stressors that cannot be avoided; and 4) providing maintenance psychopharmacologic treatment to individuals at risk for recurrences. For maximal progress, all four strategies should be used concomitantly. The last-mentioned also requires a paradigm shift among clinicians (see Chapter 6, this volume).

Frequent Recurrences

As shown in Figure 1–3 and described by many researchers (Angst et al. 1973; Greden 2000; Grof et al. 1973; Judd et al. 2000; Maj et al. 1992; Pine et al. 1998), undetected and untreated subclinical

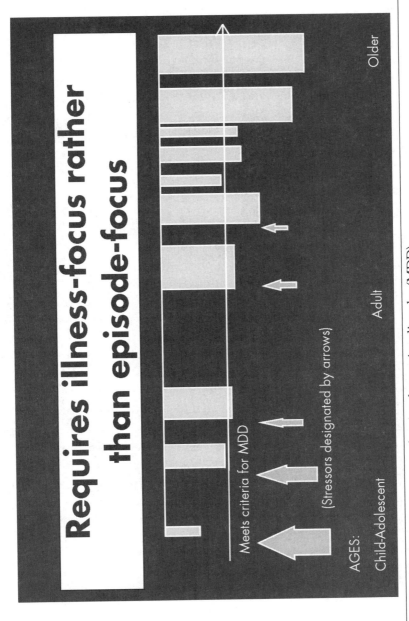

Figure 1–3. Longitudinal course of major depressive disorder (MDD).

depressive symptoms usually progress to full-fledged depressive episodes during subsequent years; the risk of new episodes increases (Pine et al. 1998), and each new episode tends to occur sooner ("cycle acceleration"), last longer, become more severe, and apparently become more difficult to treat, perhaps leading to treatment-resistant depression (see also Chapter 3 in this volume).

As described in Chapter 6 of this book, earlier detection, earlier effective intervention, and stringent protection of wellness may be essential for preventing recurrences of MDD and reducing its horrendous burden. If we fail to do this, frightening neurobiological cascades may begin to develop that accentuate the disabilities and burdens resulting from MDD.

Inadequate Emphasis on Recurrence Prevention

Because the evidence is strong that MDD recurrences are the norm when antidepressant maintenance treatment is not provided, and that the consequences of such recurrences are profound, it is perplexing that clinicians have not paid more attention to maintenance studies and treatments.

Twentieth-century concepts of depression failed to emphasize longitudinal course. Childhood depression was considered nonexistent; clinicians were taught that MDD had its onset predominantly during middle age, and clinicians were not taught to consider that mild subclinical symptoms were often early, less-severe stages of a lifetime disorder (Greden 2000). Use of different diagnostic terms—MDD versus dysthymia— encouraged the concept that the milder form was not prodromal for the more severe forms of the disorder. There was lack of understanding about how stress and genetic vulnerabilities are intertwined. When stressors were present—usually the case at least in the earlier stages of the disorder—the designation of "reactive" depression was overemphasized. Treatment pressures were on discontinuing medications after subjective improvement rather than maintaining them to help the patient cope with the next unavoidable stress and the next recurrence. The absence of laboratory tests still makes it difficult to identify patients at high risk for recurrences. Long-term studies were not emphasized, and funds for them were scarce. Lack of enthusiasm about the modest effectiveness of the earliest antidepressants (e.g., Prien et al. 1973, 1984) produced a dampening influence. Only retrospectively did we learn that the prevailing pattern of lowering medication dosages to inadequate maintenance levels may have been responsible for such modest results and that full antidepressant doses may have been necessary. Financial pressures associated with the costs of newer antidepressants have joined the list of reasons that discourage clinicians from recommending extended antidepressant maintenance. Finally, ever-present stigma interferes with accurate diagnosis, prescription patterns, and adherence to maintenance treatment.

The sands are shifting. During the past decade, recommendations for indefinite and even lifetime maintenance treatment for individuals at high risk for recurrences have been more frequent (Greden 1992, 1993). Disease management pathways and treatment guidelines are gradually incorporating longer durations of maintenance treatment for those with recurrences or chronic depression. (In my judgment, they remain too short.) Studies on the long-term effectiveness of antidepressant medications continue to be conducted, and the evidence is statistically significant and strikingly consistent. Longer-term research projects, such as the National Institute of Mental Health–funded STAR*D multicenter project, are assessing sequential steps for overcoming treatment-resistant depression. Pharmaceutical industry participation in longer-term maintenance studies also has generated valuable data (Keller et al. 2000). Considering the magnitude of disability that results from depression, however, the funding for long-term studies from all sources remains insufficient.

Poor Maintenance Treatment Adherence and Stigma

In addition to clinicians' lack of awareness and lack of prescription of extended maintenance medication, poor adherence to treatment among patients is a major problem (Crisp et al. 2000). Poor adherence is often driven by prevailing stigma about depression. Various estimates suggest the following:

- Fewer than 10% of individuals with MDD have ever seen a psychiatrist.
- 10%–20% of individuals whose disorders have been diagnosed as depression state that they do not want an antidepressant.
- Approximately 1 in 5 MDD patients do not fill their first antidepressant prescription.
- Only about half of patients who fill their first antidepressant prescription continue to take the drug after 5–6 months (Katon et al. 1999).

If we are to ever succeed in improving MDD treatment, the problems of late detection, underdiagnosis, undertreatment, and avoidance of maintenance must be overcome. If improved adherence to treatment is to occur, we must concomitantly attack the worldwide stigma associated with depression.

There are indications that we are making progress, with celebrities, corporate leaders, politicians, and men in general appearing more ready to acknowledge their depression (e.g., Wartick 2000). The U.S. Surgeon General made depression and related mental health issues *the* national health priority, stating, "There's no scientific reason to differentiate between mental health and other kinds of health. Mental illnesses are physical illnesses" (Satcher 2000). Enhanced knowledge and newer, more effective treatments are essential in our attack on depression, but decreased stigma and better adherence are just as essential.

Brain Tissue Degeneration

During the past few years, exciting neuroscience investigations have unveiled new findings on the mechanisms of neuronal production, growth, and destruction, emphasizing the effects that chronic stress and elevated stress hormones (glucocorticoids) have on brain tissue and neuronal structure. Investigators have learned the following:

- A substantial number of new granule neurons are produced in the dentate gyrus throughout the development cycle, even in adulthood (Gould et al. 2000).

- Adult neurogenesis represents a distinctive form of structural plasticity that can be regulated by the environment (Gould et al. 2000).
- New neurons play an important role in hippocampal function (the area that has been studied most to date).
- Repeated stress causes shortening and debranching of dendrites in the CA3 region of the hippocampus, suppresses neurogenesis (McEwen 2000), and leads to neuronal atrophy and cell death (Duman et al. 2000).
- Hippocampal dysfunction resulting from such neuronal degeneration may play a role in the symptoms of MDD (McEwen 2000) and perhaps its recurrent pattern.
- Other brain regions may also be affected (McEwen 2000).

The mechanisms that interfere with neurogenesis and produce brain neuronal degeneration are complex, involving 1) interactions among glucocorticoids, excitatory amino acids, and neurotransmitters such as serotonin (McEwen 2000); 2) interactions and cascades among brain neurotransmitters, the cyclic adenosine monophosphate (cAMP) system, and brain neurotrophins such as brain-derived neurotrophic factor (BDNF), neurotrophic growth factor (NGF), or *bcl-2* (Duman et al. 2000); and 3) exposure to environmental toxins such as alcohol or drugs and/or toxic events such as brain hypoxia from sleep apnea or circulatory problems (Sapolsky 2000).

Of relevance to depression, MDD episodes are often precipitated by stressors (Kendler et al. 1999). In addition, the episodes themselves are stressors; they are associated with chronic, low-grade hypersecretion of glucocorticoids and often coexist with medical conditions or substance abuse. This constellation is an incubator for neuronal degeneration. Thus, it is not surprising that the study of neuronal degeneration has moved from the basic to the clinical arena. Sheline et al. (1996) used magnetic resonance imaging (MRI) assessments of hippocampal structure to compare women with severe, chronic depression with age- and sex-matched control subjects and found evidence of hippocampal atrophy in those with depression, with the major predictor being the number of days spent depressed in one's lifetime. Postmortem observations support these brain imaging findings (Manji et al. 2000).

Although many details remain to be clarified, there is a validity to the mechanisms, with recurrent episodes of depression appearing to lead to a greater number of days spent with depression, meaning more days with chronic sustained elevations of glucocorticoids bathing the brain, lower levels of neurotrophins, greater vulnerability to toxins, and evolving brain degeneration. For clinical, social, and financial reasons, the message has long been that it is important to treat MDD adequately to the point of remission, to sustain wellness, and to prevent recurrences. Now we have data suggesting that not doing this launches a cascade of brain damage.

We have reason to hope that destructive brain processes might be averted or even reversible. Lithium has been demonstrated to robustly increase the expression of *bcl-2*, thus not only exerting neuroprotective effects but also enhancing hippocampal neurogenesis, and valproate has been demonstrated to robustly promote neurite outgrowth (Manji et al. 2000). In a follow-up clinical study, Moore et al. (2000) demonstrated a pharmacological increase in human brain gray matter in a structural MRI study of patients with mood disorders. These data support a reconceptualization of the optimal long-term treatment of recurrent depression, raising the prospect that such treatment may be aided by earlier use of agents with neurotrophic/neuroprotective effects, even for individuals with unipolar depression. This would constitute a paradigm shift for most clinicians.

Strategies to Prevent Recurrences and Reduce the Burden of MDD

Modifications to our current approaches are required if we are to reduce the disability resulting from MDD. Good beginning points constitute the topics of this book.

Clinicians need to recognize and respond to the needs of special populations and clinical high-risk groups, including the following:

- Women during high-risk periods in their reproductive cycle throughout their life spans (see Chapter 2)

- Individuals who already have developed chronic and recurrent depression, a group for which clinicians may especially wish to emphasize combinations of antidepressants and psychotherapy (see Chapter 3)
- Individuals with bipolar disorder, emphasizing the complete array of new and old treatment modalities in new and old combinations (see Chapter 4)
- Clinicians must also incorporate new treatment strategies as they are developed, such as minimally invasive brain stimulation for treatment of resistant and recurrent depression (see Chapter 5).
- Clinicians need to shift the emphasis in their approach to recurrent depression, prioritizing the *prevention* of recurrences and using all methods shown to make a difference.

This last-mentioned topic, in essence a "call to arms," is addressed throughout this book, with the final chapter summarizing 12 essential steps to be integrated into clinical practice (see Chapter 6). If such a call to arms were to be launched, MDD would not necessarily retain its inglorious position as being among the world's leading disorders in producing disability and burden.

References

Angst J, Baastrup P, Grof P, et al: The course of monopolar depression and bipolar psychoses. Psychiatria Neurolgia, Neurochirurgia 76: 489–500, 1973

Berndt ER, Koran LM, Finkelstein SN, et al: Lost human capital from early onset chronic depression. Am J Psychiatry 157:940–947, 2000

Crisp AH, Gelder MG, Rix S, et al: Stigmatisation of people with mental illness. Br J Psychiatry 177:4–7, 2000

Duman RS, Malberg J, Nakagawa S, et al: Neuronal plasticity and survival in mood disorders. Biol Psychiatry 48:732–739, 2000

Fisher LM: The race to cash in on the genetic code. New York Times. August 29, 1999

Ghaziuddin N, King CA, Welch KB, et al: Serotonin dysregulation in adolescents with major depression: hormone response to meta-chlorophenylpiperazine (mCPP) infusion. Psychiatry Res 95:183–194, 2000

Gould E, Tanapat P, Rydel T, et al: Regulation of hippocampal neurogenesis in adulthood. Biol Psychiatry 48:715–720, 2000

Greden JF: Recurrent Depression—A Lifetime Disorder: Audioconference for Family Practice Physicians in the Midwest (videocassette). Indianapolis, IN, Dista Products (Eli Lilly and Co), 1992

Greden, JF: Antidepressant maintenance medications: when to discontinue and how to stop. J Clin Psychiatry 54:39–45, 1993

Greden JF: Antidepressant maintenance medications, in Pharmacotherapy for Mood, Anxiety, and Cognitive Disorders. Edited by Halbreich U, Montgomery S. Washington, DC, American Psychiatric Press, 2000, pp 315–330

Grof P, Angst J, Haines T: The clinical course of depression: practical issues, in Classification and Prediction of Outcome of Depression. Edited by Angst J. New York, FK Schattauer Verlag, 1973, pp 141–155

Hirschfeld RM, Keller MB, Panico S, et al: The National Depressive and Manic-Depressive Association consensus statement on the undertreatment of depression. JAMA 277:333–340, 1997

Judd LL, Paulus M, Schettler P, et al: Does incomplete recovery from first lifetime major depressive episode herald a chronic course of illness? Am J Psychiatry 157:1501–1504, 2000

Kamlet M, Paul N, Greenhouse J, et al: Cost utility analysis of maintenance treatment for recurrent depression. Control Clin Trials 16:17–40, 1993

Katon W, Von Korff M, Lin E, et al: Stepped collaborative care for primary care patients with persistent symptoms of depression: a randomized trial. Arch Gen Psychiatry 56:1109–1115, 1999

Keller MB, McCullough JP, Klein DN, et al: A comparison of nefazodone, the cognitive behavioral-analysis system of psychotherapy, and their combination for the treatment of chronic depression. N Engl J Med 342:1462–1470, 2000

Kendler KS, Kessler RC, Neale MC, et al: The prediction of major depression in women: toward an integrated etiologic model. Am J Psychiatry 150:1139–1148, 1993a

Kendler KS, Neale MC, Kessler RC, et al: A longitudinal twin study of 1-year prevalence of major depression in women. Arch Gen Psychiatry 50:843–852, 1993b

Kendler KS, Karkowski LM, Prescott CA: Causal relationship between stressful life events and the onset of major depression. Am J Psychiatry 156:837–841, 1999

Kessler RC, McGonagle KA, Swartz M, et al: Sex and depression in the National Comorbidity Survey. I: lifetime prevalence, chronicity and recurrence. J Affect Disord 29:85–96, 1993

Kessler RC, McGonagle KA, Zhao S, et al: Lifetime and 12-month prevalence of DSM-III-R psychiatric disorders in the United States: results from the National Comorbidity Survey. Arch Gen Psychiatry 51:8–19, 1994

Klein DN, Schatzberg AF, McCullough JP, et al: Age of onset in chronic major depression: relation to demographic and clinical variables, family history, and treatment response. J Affect Disord 55:149–157, 1999

Koch, W: Senate panel hears stories of suicide's tragedy, stigma. USA Today, February 9, 2000, A18

Lopez JF, Chalmers DT, Little KY, et al: Regulation of serotonin 1a, glucocorticoid, and mineralocorticoid receptor in rat and human hippocampus: implications for the neurobiology of depression. Biol Psychiatry 43:547–573, 1998

Maj M, Veltro F, Pirozzi R, et al: Pattern of recurrence of illness after recovery from an episode of major depression: a prospective study. Am J Psychiatry 149:795–800, 1992

Manji HK, Moore GJ, Chen G: Clinical and preclinical evidence for the neurotrophic effects of mood stabilizers: implications for the pathophysiology and treatment of manic-depressive illness. Biol Psychiatry 48:740–754, 2000

McEwen BS: Effects of adverse experiences for brain structure and function. Biol Psychiatry 48:721–731, 2000

Mintz J, Mintz LI, Arruda MJ, et al: Treatment of depression and the functional capacity of work. Arch Gen Psychiatry 49:761–768, 1992

Moore GJ, Bebchuk JM, Wilds IB, et al: Lithium-induced increase in human brain grey matter. Lancet 356:1241–1242, 2000

Murray, CJL, Lopez AD: The Global Burden of Disease: A Comprehensive Assessment of Mortality and Disability from Disease, Injuries, and Risk Factors in 1990 and Projected to 2020, Vol 1. Cambridge, MA, Harvard University Press, 1996

Pfeffer C: The Suicidal Child. New York, Guilford, 1986

Pfeffer CR: Prevention of youth suicide (editorial). New York State Journal of Medicine 92:85–86, 1992

Pine DS, Cohen P, Gurley D, et al: The risk for early adulthood anxiety and depressive disorders in adolescents with anxiety and depressive disorders. Arch Gen Psychiatry 55:56–64, 1998

Prien RF, Klett CJ, Caffey EM Jr: Lithium carbonate and imipramine in prevention of affective episodes. A comparison in recurrent affective illness. Arch Gen Psychiatry 29:420–425, 1973

Prien RF, Kupfer DJ, Mansky PA, et al: Drug therapy in the prevention of recurrences in unipolar and bipolar affective disorders. Report of the NIMH Collaborative Study Group comparing lithium carbonate, imipramine, and a lithium carbonate–imipramine combination. Arch Gen Psychiatry 41:1096–1104, 1984

Roy-Byrne P, Post RM, Uhde TW, et al: The longitudinal course of recurrent affective illness: life chart data from research patients at the NIMH. Acta Psychiatr Scand Suppl 317:5–34, 1985

Sapolsky RM: The possibility of neurotoxicity in the hippocampus in major depression: a primer on neuron death. Biol Psychiatry 48:755–765, 2000

Satcher D: From the Surgeon General. JAMA 284:950, 2000

Sheline Y, Wang P, Gado M, et al: Hippocampal atrophy in recurrent major depression. Proc Natl Acad Sci U S A 93:3908–3913, 1996

Wartick N: Depression comes out of hiding. The New York Times, June 25, 2000

Zimmer C: Chronic stress induced alterations of the HPA and serotonin receptor system in female animals: Modulation by antidepressants and estrogen. Unpublished doctoral dissertation, University of Michigan, Ann Arbor, 2000

Chapter 2

Recurrent Depression in Women Throughout the Life Span

Sheila M. Marcus, M.D.
Heather A. Flynn, Ph.D.
Elizabeth A. Young, M.D.
Neera Ghaziuddin, M.D.
Sharon Mudd, M.S., R.N., C.S., N.P.

Depression impacts an astounding 20%–23% of women at some point in their lives, thus qualifying as one of the most common public health problems in the world (Kessler et al. 1994b). This high prevalence in women is probably multifactorial, involving a complex interplay of genetic, neuroendocrine, psychosocial, and stress factors (Bifulco et al. 1998; Heim and Nemeroff 1999). In this chapter, we examine the impact of gender on recurrent major depressive disorder (MDD), emphasizing the clinical features and treatment of the illness during three key periods of hormone transition: adolescence, pregnancy and the postpartum period, and the menopausal period. Clinical features and sex differences are described first, followed by a focus on recurrences and strategies for prevention.

Depression in Adolescence

During adolescence, the sex-specific vulnerability to depression is manifested. It was once believed that adolescents do not develop depression and that the tumultuous moods of adolescence routinely normalize with age. Longitudinal studies unveiled the erroneous nature of this view (Pine et al. 1999). Because it has been misunderstood and neglected, adolescent depression is a relatively new, and long overdue, area of study.

Prevalence

Beginning in adolescence, women suffer from a higher prevalence of depression than men. A female to male ratio of 2:1 generally has been reported, but even higher ratios such as 4:1 have been reported in some communities (Olsson 1998). Epidemiological studies have suggested a prevalence rate of MDD of 4.7% among the general adolescent population and 27% among adolescents hospitalized on a psychiatric inpatient unit (Kashani and Sherman 1988). High MDD prevalence rates have also been reported among medically ill adolescents, whose depression often is undiagnosed or who often receive inappropriate treatment.

The lifetime prevalence of depressive symptoms increases with age. Many adolescents whose symptoms do not meet DSM-IV-TR criteria for the diagnosis of MDD may have subclinical features or "partial" MDD syndrome (American Psychiatric Association 2000). The prevalence of this partial syndrome may be as high as 20.7% in the past year (Cooper and Goodyer 1993). Such "moodiness" is routinely viewed as normal adolescent development and is left untreated despite data revealing that subclinical symptoms strongly predict adult major depression and confer a twofold to threefold greater risk for adult depression (Pine et al. 1999). Early-onset major depression is associated with higher rates of recurrence, comorbid disorders, and psychiatric hospitalizations (Klein et al. 1999). For women, early onset is particularly problematic. According to Berndt et al. (2000), 12%–18% of women with early onset had lower educational attainment and lower annual earnings. Appropriate and early detection and intervention for MDD in adolescent girls are critical to minimize recurrence and secondary morbidity.

Etiology

Because sex differences in depression prevalence emerge at about age 12, at the onset of puberty, it has been inferred that these differences are associated with both biological and psychosocial transitions. Both onset of menstruation (Patton et al. 1996) and Tanner staging of III or greater are associated with a higher incidence of depression in girls (Angold et al. 1999). The effect of gonadal hormones on the evolution of depression among girls, however, is not clear. Estrogen modulates a number of neurotransmitter systems involved in mood regulation, such as serotonin, norepinephrine, and corticotrophin-releasing hormone (CRH) and is closely linked to the regulatory cascade involving serotonin and stress glucocorticoids (Vamvakopoulos and Chrousos 1993). This supports the view that gonadal hormones may play an etiological role in adolescent-onset depression, perhaps in gene expression, despite data that fail to demonstrate abnormalities in circulating hormone levels in girls and women with depression.

In general, studies of the behavioral effects of estrogen suggest that it acts as an anxiolytic and promotes changes in brain serotonin (5HT) systems, similar to the effects seen with antidepressants (Altemus and Kagan 1999). Thus estrogen is not likely to cause depression. Although isolated and anecdotal reports suggest that progesterone may worsen mood, the data do not generically support the idea that progesterone causes depression or exacerbates mood symptoms (Yonkers and Bradshaw 1999). We are left with an apparent paradox: although ovarian steroids appear to help mood, the onset of increased vulnerability to depression begins at puberty. One possible explanation might be sex-specific vulnerability factors that are modulated by steroid hormones. For example, Prescott et al. (2000) examined same-sex and opposite-sex twins and found that depression is equally heritable in men and women, but that genetic vulnerability factors appear to be different for men and women. Gonadal hormones may be related to differences in how males and females react to stress. Girls may be more susceptible than boys to family discord, lack of intimacy in the family, and dysfunctional parenting style (Davies and Windle 1997). Attainment of physical maturity, dissatisfaction with weight, and increase in developmental pressures related to sexuality may be variables that influence depression onset at this developmental stage. When it occurs, sexual abuse may be a devastating stressor leading to later depression (Bifulco et al. 1998), even involving long-term dysregulation of the hypo-thalamic-pituitary-adrenal (HPA) axis (Heim and Nemeroff 1999).

It is puzzling that whereas the onset of puberty marks a higher prevalence of depression among Caucasian girls in the United States, this association has not been found in some studies of African American or Hispanic girls (Hayward et al. 1999). Mexican American and African American adolescents may be at a greater risk for depression than Americans of Chinese descent (Chen et al. 1997; Roberts et al. 1997). Therefore, there appears to be a complex interaction between ethnicity and sociocultural factors in the ex-pression of depression. In some societies, depressive syndrome is not recognized as an illness and there is no concept for it in the cul-tural schema (Castillo 1997). Clinicians need to be aware of the dif-ference in reporting styles of emotional distress and possible taboos against acknowledging the need for treatment when they are treating patients from diverse cultural backgrounds.

Clinical Features

Common symptoms of adolescent depression are irritability, hopelessness, anhedonia, changes in sleep and appetite, aca-demic decline, reduced energy, reduced social interactions, so-matic symptoms, and suicidal ideation. Depressed adolescents display many signs and symptoms of depression noted among adults, but there are several important age- and sex-related dif-ferences in the presentation of adolescent depression. Therefore, sex and developmental factors should be taken into consider-ation during the evaluation of a depressed adolescent. Girls, for instance, may be more likely than boys to admit to internalizing symptoms such as depression and anxiety (Ostrov et al. 1989). Girls are also more likely to report somatic symptoms such as headaches and to attempt suicide, but with less lethality per at-tempt. Denial of depression, common among adolescents, may be more frequently encountered in adolescent boys than girls. Ir-ritability is a common presenting symptom and may be reported as a "short fuse," with trivial incidents resulting in major reac-tions. A pervasive sense of boredom may indicate an underlying dysregulation of the dopaminergic pleasure system. Depressed adolescents may report difficulty in getting along with their families and peers. Common hallmark neurovegetative symptoms such as insomnia and anorexia may be absent in some depressed adolescents, while many report atypical symptoms such as hypersomnia and increased appetite (Kaminski et al. 1995).

Physical symptoms such as headache and stomach pain are common presenting complaints in adolescents with depression (Hymas et al. 1996). Sadly, the depressive etiology is often overlooked by clinicians unfamiliar with this age group—a lost opportunity for early diagnosis. Egger et al. (1998) reported that although somatic complaints may be associated with depression, few adolescents who presented with these complaints were likely to receive a psychiatric evaluation. Headaches may be more commonly associated with internalizing disorders such as depression and anxiety in girls and with externalizing disorders such as conduct disorder in boys.

Substance abuse is a common problem among adolescents with depression. The association with substance abuse is complex, and adolescents with early-onset depression are at increased risk for alcohol abuse and dependence. Likewise, early-onset alcoholism is related to other serotonergic abnormalities (Johnson et al. 2000) and has a reported association with the long allele of the serotonin (5-HT) transporter. There is also an important association between depression and cigarette smoking, particularly in girls. Boys and girls who smoke cigarettes are twice as likely to develop depression as their nonsmoking peers, with the association strongest in girls (Choi et al. 1997; Olsson 1998).

Anxiety and obsessive symptoms have been observed in many adolescents with depression. One study found that the symptom of anxiety exerts an independent and additive effect on suicidality; therefore, depressed adolescents with symptoms of anxiety may be more suicidal (Ghaziuddin et al. 2000). Anxiety may also be expressed in somatic symptoms, such as frequent headaches and other physical complaints.

Complications

Suicide

Many adverse sequelae result when depression is inadequately treated during adolescence. Of these, suicide is the most devastating. It is the second leading cause of death among adolescents (National Center for Health Statistics 1990), and suicidal behavior is the most common psychiatric emergency during adolescence (Robinson 1986).

Sex differences in the rates and methods of suicide attempts and completion are marked during adolescence and suggest the importance of studying risk factors independently for boys and girls. Although adolescent girls attempt suicide more frequently than boys, the ratio of male to female completed suicides among 15- to 24-year-olds is approximately 5:1 (National Center for Health Statistics 1990). Sex differences have also been noted in the method of suicide attempts. Firearms are the most common method of completed suicide during adolescence; however, females are much more likely than males to attempt and commit suicide via self-poisoning (Berman and Jobes 1991). Psychiatric management of all adolescents who attempt suicide should include education of the patient and parents regarding issues relevant to gun availability, gun safety, and storage of medications that have the potential to be used for self-poisoning.

Psychosocial

Other commonly reported complications associated with depression include lack of satisfying social relationships, academic decline, and a possible association with teenage pregnancy (Dolgan 1990). These psychosocial sequelae, coupled with risk of recurrent depression and secondary morbidity, speak to the importance of adequate treatment during adolescence.

Treatment

General Issues

Treatment of adolescent depression usually includes a combination of psychotherapy and pharmacotherapy. Mild depression conventionally is treated with psychotherapy alone. Cognitive-behavioral therapy (CBT) and social skills groups may be useful preventive strategies. The impact of brief intervention strategies, such as education and stress management, as a prevention technique for adolescents who are at risk for depression is an area of promising research; these strategies have been effective in adult women.

Nonadherence (a term preferable to *noncompliance*) with treatment is a major issue among adolescents. It should be considered in adolescents whose depression is treatment resistant. Ghaziuddin et al. (1999) found that 40% of adolescents do not follow through with medication recommendations given at the time of discharge from an inpatient unit. Sex differences regarding treatment adherence are not known. Sensitivity to negative peer influences regarding medication and concern about weight gain are important issues that may negatively impact treatment adherence in girls. In boys, greater denial of depression to preserve the "tough male" stereotype may impact depression detection and treatment.

The current generation of adolescents, who have grown up during the explosive growth of the selective serotonin reuptake inhibitors (SSRIs) and who have witnessed increased emphasis on direct pharmaceutical marketing, public programs addressing MDD, and depression education on the Internet, may be less vulnerable than previous generations to stigmatization. It is hoped that increased public awareness and gradual destigmatization of MDD will increase access to appropriate treatment strategies, enhance adherence with necessary therapies, improve outcomes, and prevent the massive burden of MDD that begins during this key developmental phase in life.

Pharmacotherapy

Scientific evidence for effective pharmacological treatment of adolescent depression is less robust than it is for treatment of adults, according to the literature. Although tricyclic antidepressants (TCAs) are known to be highly effective in the treatment of adult depression, these agents generally have been found to be ineffective for the treatment of depressed adolescents (Geller et al. 1990; Ryan et al. 1986; Strober et al. 1990). SSRIs, specifically fluoxetine, may be more effective than TCAs in treating depressed adolescents (Jain et al. 1992). Although SSRIs may be comparable, fluoxetine is one of the few SSRIs that has been systematically evaluated in children and adolescents. In a randomized, placebo-controlled study, 56% of children (ages 7–17) with MDD improved significantly when treated with fluoxetine (20 mg/day) administered over an 8-week period (Emslie et. al 1997). The possibility that response to treatment with SSRIs may differ among children, adolescents, and adults remains to be tested. If so, different strategies must be developed for any age group whose depression remains treatment resistant.

Summary

Depression is a common disorder in both boys and girls, but occurs more frequently among adolescent girls. Even though the onset of symptoms that ultimately evolve into lifetime major depressive illness often occurs during adolescence, the illness is frequently not recognized or treated for many years, sometimes even decades. Lack of recognition contributes to secondary morbidity and recurrence. This is of particular concern in young women who may have negative functional outcomes and disturbance in their intimate relationships (Rao et al. 1999). Comorbid illnesses, such as alcohol dependence and simple and social phobia, further complicate depression when it occurs early in the life span. Whether this is the result of underlying abnormalities or developmental aspects is unknown, but the net impact is that adolescent MDD may represent a more malignant form of the disorder (Alpert et al. 1999). Other, more subtle outcomes, which are difficult to measure, may include lack of satisfying relationships, inability to reach full academic potential, and difficulty in assuming adult responsibilities at desired times. Lacking true preventive approaches, we need to emphasize effective outreach to better detect depression, treat it effectively in adolescence, and prevent secondary morbidities during this crucial phase in the female life span.

Jenny developed symptoms of depression shortly after her parents' divorce when she was 16. Her symptoms were relatively mild and included academic decline, irritability, complaints of feeling bored, diminished energy, and frequent headaches. Although Jenny experienced some episodes of low mood and minor symptoms of anxiety; she did not reveal these to her mother or friends and received no medical attention. Her mother later reflected that her own mood symptoms and preoccupation with circumstances of her divorce may have contributed to underrecognition of her daughter's distress. Jenny's minor symptoms improved after about 6 months. During the remainder of high school, she had no further depression, but did fail a speech class because she was unable to perform public speaking. Jenny entered college at age 18, and depression reemerged during the fall term. She attributed this to her stressful academic schedule and separation from home. Jenny returned home after the first term and resumed college the following fall at a small community college closer to home. At age 24, following a broken relationship, she experienced an episode of depression that met DSM-IV-TR criteria for MDD. Even then, her MDD was not diagnosed.

Jenny's case is fairly typical of adolescent depression in that minor symptoms and somatic complaints were not recognized at the time of presentation and her depression remained untreated. In Jenny's case, concurrent maternal illness and the stress of parental divorce may have complicated the presentation and contributed to underdetection, but such circumstances are common. Comorbid anxiety disorder further complicated her illness and resulted in academic decline and a suboptimal adjustment to college.

Depression in Pregnancy and the Postpartum Period

Prevalence

Pregnancy and the postpartum period are times of particular vulnerability to depression. As with adolescence, a changing hormone milieu plays a role in the onset of depressive episodes. It was once thought that high levels of estrogen and progesterone during pregnancy created a "honeymoon" period for affective illness. More recent studies suggest that the prevalence of depression during pregnancy (10%) is identical to that in nongravid women (Cohen et al. 1998). Rapidly falling progesterone and estrogen levels, coupled with the sensitizing effect of high prolactin and oxytocin, may play a role in the substantial increase in depression following delivery. Thyroid dysfunction may also play a role. Rates of hypothyroidism in the postpartum period are estimated to be as high as 9% (Althshuler et al. 1998). Studies of the prevalence of postpartum depression suggest that it occurs after 10%–15% of all deliveries, making it one of the most common complications of pregnancy (Wisner et al. 1996). Although it is well established that depression is a recurrent disorder, few studies have been conducted on the specific risk of recurrence of unipolar illness during pregnancy or its relationship to medication withdrawal at the time of conception. Additionally, blood levels of antidepressants fall during late pregnancy (Altshuler et al. 1998) and may predispose women to relapse even if they are still taking medication.

Recurrence of MDD following childbirth in women with previous depression is high, with estimates ranging from 25% to 50% (Wisner et al. 1996). In women with bipolar illness, the risk of postpartum relapse is also well-established and estimated to be between 30% and 50%, particularly when mood stabilizers are discontinued (Cohen et al. 1995). Viguera et al. (2000) found that the rate of recurrence of bipolar illness in pregnant women was 52% during the 40 weeks following conception when lithium was discontinued. The risk of relapse is particularly high for women who have had episodes of depressive illness with psychotic features. Whereas the initial risk of postpartum psychosis is estimated to be 0.1%–0.2% (Kumar and Robson 1984), the risk of recurrence of puerperal psychosis after an index episode is estimated to be 75%–90% (Altshuler et al. 1998). Pregnancy and the months following delivery pose a particular threat of recurrent illness in women with a history of mood disorders. Vigilance is mandatory in caring for these patients.

Risk Factors

As during other times, risk of depression during pregnancy and the postpartum period is influenced by genetic vulnerability and stressful life events. A number of studies have examined risk factors for the occurrence of depression in pregnant and lactating women. In a screening study among a large sample of women at the University of Michigan Health System, factors such as previous depression, single marital status, poor health functioning, and drinking during pregnancy emerged as risk factors for depression in the prenatal period (Marcus et al. 2000). Other studies have produced similar findings and have suggested that personal and family history of mood disorder, marital conflict, younger age, and limited social support, along with a greater number of children, are also risk factors for depression during pregnancy (O'Hara 1986).

Clinical Features

DSM-IV-TR criteria for MDD overlap with many symptoms of pregnancy itself. Changes in appetite and sleep, and fatigue and diminished energy, are common. These symptoms result in uncertainty about prevalence and course of depression during pregnancy. The majority of women who present to medical practitioners with symptoms of depression do so in the primary care or obstetric setting. Often this overlap of symptomatology, the rapid pace of primary care appointments, and a woman's reluctance to disclose symptoms make detection and treatment of depression difficult during pregnancy.

DSM-IV-TR defines depression with postpartum onset as MDD that begins within the first 4 weeks following delivery. The literature on prevalence is problematic (Altshuler et al. 1998). As during pregnancy, reluctance to admit to having depressive symptoms during a time many women expect to be enjoyable, as well as inconsistencies in the time frame used to define postpartum illness, creates uncertainty. Symptoms of postpartum depression include those of MDD, but many have prominent features of anxiety. Additionally, insecurity about capacity to parent and recurrent ruminations about the health and well-being of the infant are common. Psychomotor agitation (e.g., pacing, nervousness) is common. Pediatricians frequently are the first to note changes in the mothers, prompted by the multiple anxious and obsessive phone calls they receive from such "nervous mothers," often about lactation and infant health.

Sequelae

Major Depression During Pregnancy

Untreated psychiatric illness can have adverse effects on both the mother and the fetus. Relapses increase the risk of chronicity and treatment resistance in depression (Greden and Tandon 1995).

Suicidality, poor nutrition, inadequate self-care, and insomnia are associated with exacerbation of depression during pregnancy and represent significant risks of not effectively treating MDD.

Significant depression is associated with low birthweight, an increased risk of premature delivery, and preeclampsia in the mother (Kurki et al. 2000; Steer et al. 1992). There are additional questions concerning the potential negative effect of untreated psychiatric disorders and elevated levels of cortisol on fetoplacental integrity and central nervous system development (Cohen and Rosenbaum 1998). The potential risks of withholding psychotropic medications during gestation, summarized by Miller (1991), include the following:

- Malnutrition, secondary to loss of appetite, motivation, or judgment
- Attempts at premature delivery
- Fetal abuse or neonaticide
- Inability to participate in prenatal care
- Precipitous delivery when the patient is unable to identify labor

Postpartum Depression

Depression in the postpartum period may have adverse consequences for both the mother and her child. The detrimental effect of postpartum depression on the mother-infant relationship and development of the child has been studied. Mothers with untreated postpartum depression display less affection and are less responsive to infant cues. Their infants perform worse on object concept tasks and demonstrate mild behavioral difficulties (Murray 1992). Longitudinal studies suggest that these poorer outcomes continue into later child development (Murray et al. 1996; Sharp et al. 1995)

Treatment

Major Depression During Pregnancy

The risks and benefits of continuing antidepressants during pregnancy must be determined by the patient and her physician on an individual basis. The decision is never simple. Many women have great difficulty balancing the risk of undertreating their illness with that of exposing their infants to medication. All pregnant women should receive support and education as they make this critical treatment decision. There are no easy answers. Although it is still common practice to withdraw medications at the time of conception, many patients with previous MDD relapse during or after pregnancy if this step is taken haphazardly.

Some women with histories of mild or subsyndromal illness may use nonpharmacologic prevention strategies during pregnancy. One recommendation is that only women with long periods of interepisode well-being should discontinue medications at the time of conception. Prepregnancy planning is essential to provide a slow medication taper, minimizing risk of recurrence of depression. Prevention strategies, such as not consuming alcohol or caffeine and not smoking, may also diminish relapse risk. Maintenance of circadian rhythm, exercise, stress management, and psychotherapy are also useful as prevention strategies and as adjunctive strategies when medications are used. Many women benefit from both interpersonal psychotherapy and CBT, which have been used to reduce risk of relapse in women with recurrent illness (Frank and Thase 1999). Mobilizing support systems may be useful for women who are separated from extended family. Coordination of care with family members and other members of the treatment team is essential to monitor symptoms and to ensure adherence to treatment, particularly when medications are used. Disclosure of information on antidepressant use during pregnancy as well as on the risk of undertreatment of illness is critical when preparing a pregnant woman and her family for medication use. Usually when symptoms are moderate to severe, when there have been recurrences, and anxiety or insomnia is prominent, antidepressant medications are indicated. Medication is essential when suicidality, inadequate nutrition, or risk-taking behavior threaten the pregnancy.

Medication choice should be guided by data supporting fetal safety (see Table 2–1). Antidepressants should be given in the lowest doses necessary to control symptoms. However, increased maternal blood volumes and accelerated renal clearance of the drugs may necessitate increasing doses in the third trimester.

Table 2–1. Teratogenicity, neonatal toxicity, and behavioral risks associated with antidepressant and mood stabilizing medication use during pregnancy and lactation

Drug	Teratogenicity	Neonatal toxicity	Developmental risks	Lactation risks
Benzodiazepines	Possibly causes cleft palate	Multiple sequelae associated with prenatal exposure, including withdrawal syndrome with sustained use in third trimester	Some evidence of developmental delay	Secreted into breastmilk; may contribute to lethargy, weight loss, and kernicterus in exposed infants
Bupropion	No adequate well-controlled studies; reproductive studies in animals at dose 7–12 times human dose revealed no evidence of teratogenicity	No information	No studies conducted	Pharmacokinetic studies have revealed that bupropion and its metabolites are secreted into breastmilk
Carbamazepine/ anticonvulsants	Increased risk of congenital malformations, neural tube defects, craniofacial anomalies, and other defects	Limited data	Difficult to determine because of confounding effects of maternal epilepsy	May be safer than lithium for breastfeeding women who require mood stabilizers
Lithium	Increased risk of cardiac congenital anomalies	Associated with neonatal morbidity; increased risk of mortality; may be associated with specific neonatal syndromes; neonatal toxicity may result when maternal blood levels are not closely monitored in third trimester and immediately postpartum	No developmental risks noted in humans	Should not be used during breastfeeding because of its toxicity

Table 2–1. Teratogenicity, neonatal toxicity, and behavioral risks associated with antidepressant and mood stabilizing medication use during pregnancy and lactation (*continued*)

Drug	Teratogenicity	Neonatal toxicity	Developmental risks	Lactation risks
Monoamine oxidase inhibitors (MAOIs)	Contraindicated in pregnancy	Contraindicated in pregnancy	Contraindicated in pregnancy	Contraindicated in lactation
Selective serotonin reuptake inhibitors (SSRIs)	Found to be safe for both mother and fetus; no increase in specific malformations in studies to date	Anecdotal reports of possible colic, irritability, and increased respiratory rate (paroxetine only)	One study found no adverse neuropsychiatric effects on language, IQ, or behavior in children up to 5 years of age (fluoxetine only)	Both fluoxetine and sertraline are secreted into breastmilk; because fluoxetine has a long half life, exposure through breastmilk may lead to detectable levels in infants; more study needed
Tricyclic agents	No congenital defects found with fetal exposure	A number of perinatal syndromes associated with withdrawal have been found	Limited data on humans; one study found no adverse neuropsychiatric effects on language, IQ, or behavior in children up to 5 years of age	Tricyclic agents are secreted into breastmilk; infants found to be at low risk for adverse effects; more study needed

Clinicians generally prefer using SSRIs and secondary amine TCAs for treatment of depression during pregnancy and lactation. Research suggests that SSRIs are safe for use in all three trimesters, with no increase in teratogenic effect and no substantial behavioral toxicity (Kulin et al.1998; Pastuszak et al. 1993; Stowe et al. 1997; Wisner et al. 1999). In a study from the Swedish Medical Birth Registry, no increase in congenital abnormalities was found in the perinatal period in 969 infants whose mothers used SSRIs and/or TCAs (Ericson et al. 1999). Information regarding behavioral toxicity is sparse, but in one study, children exposed to fluoxetine and TCAs were similar to sibling control subjects in IQ, language development, and behavioral development, when followed through the age of 86 months (Nulman et al. 1997).

TCAs have a lengthy history of use in pregnancy. A review of the literature from 1966 to 1995 did not identify any associations between fetal exposure to TCAs and rates of congenital malformation in 414 cases of first trimester exposure (Altshuler et al. 1996). There have been anecdotal reports of infant withdrawal, including irritability, respiratory difficulty, and seizures, during the neonatal period (Wisner and Perel 1996). Limited data exist on bupropion and venlafaxine use during pregnancy, which typically are not medications of first choice during gestation. However, when women are already taking bupropion or venlafaxine in the first trimester, it is usually best to continue these medications, rather than exposing the patients to the risk of recurrence of depression or to yet another medication, even if the latter has been better studied (Cohen 2000).

Benzodiazepines are usually contraindicated in the first trimester because of the risk of cleft palate (Altshuler et al. 1996). When anxiety is disabling and not ameliorated by antidepressants, benzodiazepines can be used intermittently during the second and third trimesters. Trazodone and diphenhydramine are often used clinically, though they are not well studied. There are limited data on the use of complementary medications and herbal remedies during pregnancy, though European studies involving *Hypericum perforatum* (St.-John's-wort) have demonstrated efficacy in treating mild-to-moderate depression (Wheatley 1997). Because many women self-medicate with herbal remedies, assuming them to be "natural," it is important to inquire about use of these agents when obtaining clinical histories of pregnant women. Table 2–2 presents U.S. Food and Drug Administration categorization of risk of psychotropic medication use during pregnancy and lactation.

Bipolar Illness During Pregnancy

Management of bipolar illness during pregnancy is complicated by demonstrated teratogenicity from the use of mood stabilizers during the first trimester. Cardiac abnormalities have been reported in the infants of women who continued to use lithium during pregnancy. The degree of risk of the most common anomaly, Ebstein's anomaly, is estimated to be 0.1%, approximately 10–20 times the rate in infants in the general population. This risk is much lower than was initially reported in the International Register of Lithium Babies (Cohen et al. 1994). Lithium use is associated with several other perinatal syndromes, including flaccidity, cyanosis, lethargy, poor sucking, and abnormal reflexes. Increases in prematurity and perinatal mortality have been reported (Wilson et al. 1983; Woody et al. 1971; Yoder et al. 1984). Prenatal exposure to valproic acid has been associated with a 1%–5% risk of neural tube defects, and the incidence of these defects in children exposed to carbamazepine is about 0.5% (Lammer et al. 1987; Lindhout et al. 1992; Omtzigt et al. 1992). Other anomalies such as hypoplastic nails and craniofacial anomalies have also been identified (Jones et al. 1989). The risks increase when multiple anticonvulsants are used concomitantly and with higher total maternal blood levels of the agents.

When women have had a long illness-free interval, mood stabilizers should be tapered slowly *before* conception to minimize the risk of exposure and recurrence. The risk of lithium exposure overall appears lower than that of other anticonvulsants, making it the mood stabilizer of choice when used in the first trimester. It is ideal, however, that none be administered during this time period. This is noteworthy given the frequency of use of valproate in clinical practice. Use of mood stabilizers during pregnancy should be preceded by a careful discussion with the woman and her family about the risks of medication exposure as well as the risks of undertreatment.

Table 2–2. U.S. FDA categorization of risk of psychotropic medication use during pregnancy and lactation

Category	Definition of risk	Psychotropic medication
A	Controlled studies show no risk to humans. Well-controlled studies in pregnant women demonstrate no risk to the fetus.	None
B	No evidence of risk in humans, but data are inadequate. Either animal studies demonstrate risk, but this has not been confirmed in human studies, or animal studies show no risk, and no well-controlled human studies have been conducted.	Bupropion* Buspirone* Clozapine* Fluoxetine* Paroxetine* Sertraline* Zolpidem*
C	Risk cannot be ruled out. Well-controlled human studies lacking. Animal studies either lacking or show risk.	Carbamazepine Chloral hydrate Citalopram Clomipramine Clonazepam Desipramine Mirtazapine Monoamine oxidase inhibitors Nefazodone Trazodone Venlafaxine

Table 2–2. U.S. FDA categorization of risk of psychotropic medication use during pregnancy and lactation *(continued)*

Category	Definition of risk	Psychotropic medication
D	Positive evidence of human fetal risk, but risk may be outweighed by potential benefit. Some evidence of risk in human studies. Drugs should be given only if potential benefit outweighs potential risk to fetus.	Alprazolam Diazepam Imipramine Lithium Nortriptyline Sodium valproate
X	Contraindicated in pregnancy. Studies in humans and/or animals show clear evidence of significant fetal risk.	Flurazepam Quazepam Temazepam Triazolam

*As listed by manufacturer.

Relapses of bipolar illness during pregnancy can be serious and should be treated aggressively with mood stabilizers and neuroleptics when clinically indicated. Lithium should be prescribed in multiple daily doses to prevent wide swings in blood levels. Doses may be increased, but the mother's level of lithium in the blood must be monitored carefully because of this increase and because renal clearance of lithium increases in the third trimester. Lithium should be reduced by as much as 30% a few weeks before delivery to avoid toxicity, which may occur following childbirth when maternal plasma volume contracts (Wisner et al. 1996). Medications initiated during pregnancy should be continued for at least 6 months following delivery to prevent postpartum relapse (Cohen et al. 1995), and possibly longer when indications are present. Women requiring mood stabilizers, particularly lithium, should be encouraged to bottlefeed their infants. Ultrasound with full fetal survey should be obtained at 16–18 weeks to assess the fetus for congenital anomalies when any mood stabilizers are used. Use of valproate or carbamazepine should be accompanied by use of folate (4 mg/day) during the first trimester (Altshuler et al. 1996).

Combination psychotherapy and pharmacotherapy is the preferred approach for treating pregnant women, whether they have unipolar or bipolar disorder.

Postpartum Depression

Decisions to use pharmacotherapy during the postpartum period should be guided primarily by the severity of past illness and current symptoms and functioning. In women with previous severe recurrent episodes, medications can be initiated during the third trimester to ensure adequate blood levels at delivery. SSRIs appear to be effective for the treatment of postpartum depression. As with all antidepressants, they are secreted into the breastmilk, with a serum-to-milk ratio of approximately 1:1. SSRIs are frequently below the threshold of detectability in assays of infant serum. Conclusions about exposure to the infant's brain should not be drawn, however, because animal studies do suggest sequestering of the drugs in the more lipophilic brain tissue (Stowe et al. 1997). There have been no substantial difficulties reported in infants of lactating mothers who used sertraline, but there are occasional reports of irritability and colic in infants exposed to fluoxetine through lactation. TCAs, similar to SSRIs, are secreted in breastmilk with a serum-to-milk ratio of approximately 1:1. TCA levels in infant plasma are variable and sometimes undetectable. Despite limited data, most studies support the use of the secondary amine TCAs (nortriptyline and desipramine) and SSRIs in lactating women (Altshuler et al. 1996).

Thyroid function testing and alcohol screening should be conducted in depressed women during pregnancy and lactation. Mobilizing support systems, encouraging family members to participate in infant feeding to prevent sleep deprivation in the mother, and ensuring proper diet and moderate exercise may be useful adjunctive treatments. Interpersonal psychotherapy may be a useful adjunctive strategy to help women adjust to the changes of motherhood (Stuart and O'Hara 1995). Suicide and infanticide are the most catastrophic outcomes of depression during pregnancy and the postpartum period. In severe, psychotic, or treatment-resistant depression, electroconvulsive therapy is considered a safe choice during pregnancy and lactation. Clinicians should not forget this option. It may be the treatment of choice when rapid intervention is essential.

Summary

The need for treatment of serious, sometimes life-threatening MDD during pregnancy and the postpartum period has been underrecognized, with potentially serious consequences for women and their children. Despite the bulk of evidence that the fetus is safe if the mother takes SSRIs or TCAs, many physicians discontinue these medications at the time of conception. The risks and consequences of this important treatment decision need to be more closely explored. Research on newer antidepressant medications, augmentation strategies, and complementary agents will add to current literature on treatment decisions that impact pregnant women.

Jill, age 24, had her first episode of depression at age 18. During the third trimester of her first pregnancy, she had intermittent periods of low mood and tearfulness, and complained of periods of "chest tightness," which were accompanied by somatic anxiety symptoms. Jill attributed these symptoms to anxiety over the impending delivery of her child. The symptoms escalated following the birth of her son. Jill couldn't understand why she felt so unhappy despite having a healthy and much-desired infant. She felt overwhelmed by her new role as a mother and was tearful and anxiously preoccupied much of the day with her son's well-being. Her constant calls to her pediatrician precipitated a referral to her own primary health care provider, who suggested a cardiac workup for her chest symptoms. Following a negative workup, a psychiatrist was consulted. A diagnosis of MDD was made. Because Jill was lactating, sertraline was initiated. Her symptoms remitted within 4 weeks, and Jill continued using medication until she became pregnant 7 months later. Because of her brief period of treatment, her previous episode, and her history of symptoms during pregnancy, a decision was made to continue her medication during the second pregnancy. She remained asymptomatic and continued the medication throughout the postpartum period, delivering a healthy daughter at term.

Depression in Midlife

Prevalence

Midlife is often considered a period of heightened risk for depression in women. Despite speculation and belief that hormonal changes cause depression in midlife, evidence to support this belief remains inconclusive (Avis et al. 1994; Kaufert et al. 1992; Nicol-Smith 1996). It could be that episodes become more severe or closer together, or that the disorder is finally diagnosed. A diathesis-stress model has been used to explain the emergence of depression in midlife (Kessler et al. 1994a). According to this model, vulnerability to depression, based on previous episodes, interacts with life stressors and role changes, which often occur in midlife, increasing susceptibility for a recurrence.

Menopause, defined as a 6-month period of amenorrhea (Holte 1998), occurs at a mean age of 50–51 years (Haynes and Parry 1998; Holte 1998). Although no direct or causal association has been found between menopause per se and depression in a number of different types of studies, some have observed an association between the transition to menopause (perimenopause) and depression. It is clear that middle-age women report a number of psychological symptoms, and these midlife years are often associated with a number of social and psychological changes. During the menopausal transition, it has been estimated that 50%–70% of women experience a variety of somatic and emotional symptoms (Schwingl et al. 1994). In clinical practice and in research studies, however, MDD is often inadequately distinguished from depressive symptoms (Rubinow et al. 1998). Moreover, depressive symptoms are often confounded by vasomotor and other associated symptoms of menopause. Accurate distinctions are critical not only for understanding the risk of onset and recurrence of depression throughout a woman's life, but also for determining the most appropriate and effective treatment options.

Several studies concluded that MDD is no more likely to occur during menopause than at any other time in a woman's life (Nolen-Hoeksema 1995a). Table 2–3 presents rates of depressive disorders diagnosed with DSM-III (American Psychiatric Association 1980) structured clinical interviews in the general population. The highest prevalence of MDD occurs between ages 25 and 44. These findings are supported by Epidemiologic Catchment Area (ECA) and National Comorbity Survey (NCS) data, showing a higher 12-month prevalence rate during the reproductive years than during the premenarchal and postmenopausal periods (Kessler et al. 1994b; Weissman et al. 1988), with the highest prevalence of MDD occurring in women in their late premenopausal years (Blazer et al. 1994; Regier et al. 1994). However, more recent data analyzed from the ECA study found a peak onset of depressive illness during the perimenopausal years (Weissman 1996).

DSM-IV-TR reports that the average age at onset for MDD is the mid-20s. Rates in men and women are highest for ages 25–44, but twice as common in adolescent and young adult women as compared with men. There is substantial evidence showing that severity and length of episodes increase as a person grows older, particularly with inadequate interepisode recovery. Findings from a number of studies support a decreased likelihood of first episode onset of depression after age 45 (Lehtinen and Joukamaa

Table 2–3. Rates of depressive disorders diagnosed with DSM-III structured clinical interviews in the general population

Age group	Female (%)	Male (%)
18–24	6.9	3.8
25–44	10.8	4.8
45–64	7.8	3.3
65+	3.2	1.2

Source. Data from Myers et al. 1984.

1994; Weissman and Olfson 1995). Avis et al. (1994) conducted a 5-year longitudinal study of the relationship between depression and menopause in women ages 45–55. After controlling for previous depression, menopausal symptoms, and hormone treatment, the authors found that the onset of menopause was not associated per se with an increased risk of depression.

Perimenopause is defined as lack of menstruation at least once during the previous 6 months and occurrence of the last menstruation less than 6 months ago. This period is associated with gradual declines in estrogen levels and may lead to an increase in depressive symptoms. This finding has led to speculation that changing estrogen levels, not low levels of estrogen associated with menopause, are responsible for mood changes in many women. A number of studies have found increases in depressive symptoms associated with perimenopause (Ballinger 1990) and with a prolonged perimenopausal period (Avis et al. 1994). Joffe et al. (1999) found that perimenopausal women were twice as likely to exhibit depressive symptoms, even after controlling for history of depression, and Joffe (2000) found that depressive symptoms were 4.6 times more likely to occur in the presence of hot flashes during the perimenopausal period.

Such studies elucidate the importance of considering a number of factors that may confound the apparent relationship of depression (at various levels) with the transition to menopause. These factors include the presence of vasomotor symptoms, sleep problems, hot flashes, and life stress; assessment of depression; and history of depression.

Etiology

It is likely that the emergence of depression during midlife in women most often represents a recurrence or relapse of a previous episode. A history of depression is strongly predictive of future episodes (Coyne et al. 1999), and severity of illness is postulated to increase with repeated exposure to stressors and previous depressive episodes (kindling) (Weiss and Post 1998). Recurrence rates of MDD have been estimated to be from 50% to 70% (Kessler et al. 1994b), and women may be more likely to experience relapse (Lewinson et al. 1989).

Some research and clinical evidence support the notion that women with a history of depression, particularly premenstrual syndrome and postpartum depression, are at an increased risk for experiencing MDD during menopause (Hay et al. 1994). Although findings are equivocal, many studies and clinical observations support the notion that women have longer recovery times from a depressive episode (Frank et al. 1988) and experience more recurrences than men. Women over age 30 may have the highest rate of recurrent depression (Ernst and Angst 1992; Kessler et al. 1994a). Because the age at onset for women typically is the early childbearing years (earlier, on average, than men), women have a longer period of exposure to recurrences. It has been speculated that depression during midlife may be the result of ongoing (as in the case of untreated, undertreated, or treatment-refractory depression) or recurrent depression. This is particularly plausible given the finding that a history of depression constitutes a major risk factor for depression in midlife.

Midlife is characterized by particular kinds of stressors and life transitions, such as children leaving home and starting their own families, loss of or caregiving of parents, occupational disruptions, marital changes, and even death of spouses or children. These kinds of changes, particularly losses and interpersonal role transitions, have been associated with onset and maintenance of depression in women (Weissman et al. 2000).

A history of depression and its interaction with these life changes may confer vulnerability for women to experience depression in the context of menopause (Kaufert et al. 1992).

The recurrent nature of depression in women, as well as the heterogeneity of biochemical functioning and sensitivity, has led to postulation about subtypes of women at risk for depression during the transition to menopause. Women at risk for depression (i.e., those who have had previous episodes) may have differential responses to hormonal changes during this period (Schmidt et al. 1998). The affective changes that may accompany fluctuation of gonadal hormones may constitute increased risk for relapse in women with a history of depression. A large body of experimental studies by Nolen-Hoeksema et al. (1995b) have found that women are significantly more likely to engage in excessive rumination in the context of depression and that rumination exacerbates the length and severity of depression. Studies have not examined the role of rumination in the onset and severity of depression in the menopausal period. The extent to which somatic, cognitive, and mood-related symptoms often associated with the transition to menopause interact with a ruminative style to initiate or exacerbate a depressive episode (particularly in patients with a history of depression) needs to be examined.

It has been theorized that the vasomotor and other somatic symptoms of perimenopause (e.g., hot flashes, night sweats, sleep disturbances) are responsible for the development of depressed mood and other problems such as fatigue, loss of energy, and concentration problems (Kronenberg 1994; Schmidt and Rubinow 1991). This theory has been supported by a few studies. Baker et al. (1996), for example, examined sleep and mood changes in premenopausal and perimenopausal women by using 1-week sleep diaries. They found that sleep and mood changes were significantly related in the perimenopausal group, but were not related in the premenopausal women. Most studies that controlled for vasomotor symptoms have not found evidence for increases in depression in the transition to menopause.

Other biological theories have been proposed, each with little conclusive evidence. It has been shown that decreasing estrogen levels may affect serotonergic activity. Studies with serotonin agonists (m-chlorophenylpiperazine [m-CPP]) have resulted in prolactin and cortisol responses (Halbreich et al. 1995). Changing levels of estrogen on serotonergic function, as well as neurotransmitter, neuroendocrine, and circadian rhythm changes (Kornstein 1997), have also been implicated in the etiology of depressive symptoms during the menopausal period.

Complicating Factors

Many symptoms of menopause, including sleep difficulties, somatic symptoms (e.g., hot flashes), fatigue, irritability, anxiety, and inability to concentrate, may overlap with symptoms of depression in women. In addition, a number of life stressors may be encountered concurrent with the transition to menopause. It is likely that many women will not recognize these symptoms as possible indicators of depression and will not seek appropriate treatment. Rather, some women may perceive these discomforts and problems as a "natural" part of aging and do not bring them to the attention of a health care provider. This is a particular concern for women who have not experienced signs and symptoms of MDD or who do not have adequate information about them. It is also likely that some health care providers do not thoroughly screen for history and symptoms of depression in women with somatic and mood complaints in the menopausal period, on the assumption that these symptoms are related to perimenopause.

Some evidence suggests the possibility that previous medication treatment for depression is related to earlier onset of menopause. Although the relationship between pharmacological treatment of depression and menopause is not known, one study found an association between antidepressant treatment for 3 years and early menopause (Harlow and Signorello 2000). This area needs further study. We recommend that previous antidepressant use be part of a comprehensive evaluation and education approach with women in the menopausal period.

Treatment

Because of the purported causal relationship between menopause and depression, hormone replacement therapy (HRT) is believed to alleviate symptoms of depression during this time. Estrogen has been postulated to produce antidepressant activity by increasing central tryptophan concentrations, enhancing catecholamine neurotransmission, reducing serotonin 5-HT$_2$ receptor binding, regulating serotonin receptor number and function, and inhibiting monoamine oxidase enzymes (Amsterdam et al. 1999; Rubinow et al. 1998). However, its usefulness as an antidepressant or as an augmentation to traditional antidepressants is inconclusive. A few studies and clinical trials suggest that estrogen alleviates depression and enhances subjective well-being (Carranza-Lira and Valentino-Figueroa 1999; Montgomery et al. 1987; Sherwin 1991). In a small double-blind, parallel-design, placebo-controlled trial of estrogen administration in perimenopausal women whose symptoms met research diagnostic criteria for depression in the absence of hot flashes, estrogen therapy was superior to placebo in reducing depressive symptomatology, including sadness, tearfulness, and social isolation (Rubinow et al. 1998). Given that the transition to menopause, more than the postmenopausal period, is associated with increased depressive symptomatology, some clinicians advocate inducing menopause through the use of a gonadotropin-releasing hormone analog, such as leuprolide, so that estrogen levels can be managed more precisely. This approach is considered in cases of severe treatment-resistant depression during perimenopause but should not be a routine approach.

Despite this evidence, when vasomotor complaints are controlled, many studies have not supported the utility of HRT in directly alleviating depression. Despite the equivocation of the evidence, Tonkelaar and Oddens (2000) studied the determinants of long-term HRT and found that mood disturbances were at least one of the reasons that HRT was initially prescribed in 53.8% of the cases and at least one of the reasons for continuation on a long-term basis (> 6 years) in 50.4% of the cases. A number of methodological limitations of studies addressing this issue may be responsible for the discrepancy between clinical belief and research, such as definition and assessment of menopausal status, identification of biochemical markers for menopause, inconsistencies in the assessment and conceptualization of depression, and statistical and methodological control of vasomotor status (Holte 1998). Because of these methodological problems, Holte (1998) suggested that recommending the use of HRT for depression in menopause is premature.

Joffe and Cohen (1998) recently reviewed treatment studies in which estrogen was used alone, as an augmentation strategy, or as a prophylactic against recurrent depression. These authors concluded that estrogen therapy alone had no benefit over placebo in the treatment of MDD. Preliminary evidence suggests that HRT may enhance response to fluoxetine, although randomized, controlled studies are needed to examine the efficacy of HRT augmentation and use of HRT as a prophylactic. Schatzberg (1998) suggested that postmenopausal women who are not taking estrogen may experience fewer side effects with TCAs and SSRIs. Brady (2000) suggested that HRT may be added as an augmentation strategy for menopausal women with depression who are not responding to antidepressants.

It is recommended that women whose symptoms meet DSM-IV-TR criteria for diagnosis of MDD, regardless of menopausal status, be treated with antidepressants and concomitant psychotherapies with demonstrated efficacy such as interpersonal therapy or CBT and that HRT not be routinely employed as the sole therapy or an alternative therapy.

> Ann, who is 47, had experienced amenorrhea for 3 months and had begun to notice seemingly unrelated symptoms such as sleep problems, irritability, sad mood, and difficulty concentrating. She attributed her symptoms to beginning menopause and to stress associated with around-the-clock caregiving of her ailing 78-year-old mother. Ann's caregiving duties had caused her to miss a great deal of work and to become isolated from her friends. Because her siblings live far from town, Ann had very little relief from taking care of her mother. Ann made an appointment with her physician to discuss the possibility of hormone replacement therapy (HRT) for menopause, because she had heard about the benefits of HRT from friends. As she discussed her symptoms with her physician, she became tearful. Ann's physician referred her to a psychiatrist, who conducted a careful assessment of current and past psychiatric functioning. The assessment revealed that Ann's symptoms met criteria for the diagnosis of MDD and that she had experienced a previous untreated episode in her mid-20s. Ann began taking an SSRI and experienced major symptom relief within 4 weeks. She was also advised to seek needed relief from caregiving duties when possible and to monitor her physical symptoms.

The Need for More Research

Effective treatments for depression do exist. Unfortunately, many women do not seek health care and some do not receive appropriate treatment. Recurrences are the rule and impact women throughout their life spans, including during adolescence, pregnancy and the postpartum period, and the menopausal period. During these periods, stressors and changing steroid hormone function act on a vulnerable genetic predisposition to illness. Undertreatment of depression then leads to more recurrences, which impact frequency and intensity of episodes later in life.

The high rates of depression recurrence in women point out the need for a comprehensive and accessible disease management approach. Screening, early intervention, pharmacologic and psychosocial interventions appropriate for women, and interventions for comorbidities must be incorporated. These strategies need to be sensitive to differing developmental issues in women throughout their life spans.

More research on depression in women is needed in the following areas:

- Appropriate pharmacologic treatments for adolescent girls, and clarification of whether sex differences are associated with different medication responsivity in young women.
- Elaboration of the relationship between glucocorticoid hormones, 5-HT, and stress at puberty and the relationship of menses and menopause to antidepressant responsivity.
- Preventive techniques for female children and adolescents with parental histories of depression to help delay or even prevent first episodes; longer term follow-up to identify brief interventions that minimize the impact of depression and risk for recurrence; genetic research strategies (e.g., genetic microarray studies) to clarify underlying complex genetic contributions to determine which individuals are candidates for early intervention to prevent MDD; determination of how psychosocial, familial, developmental, medical, and hormonal factors affect the rapid increase in depression in adolescent girls to help formulate more prevention measures.

- Mechanisms to improve adherence to medication treatment in women throughout their life spans to decrease and even prevent recurrences; identification of factors that affect treatment adherence (e.g., women who engage in rumination in response to depression are more likely to be passive and less likely to take active steps to improve their mood [Nolen-Hoeksema 1995b]); education of the public about depression to help reduce stigma and thereby encourage individuals to seek appropriate treatment; development of messages targeted to specific groups to increase medication treatment adherence (e.g., patients who are concerned about weight gain or sexual dysfunction).
- Determination of why physicians routinely discontinue medications at time of conception; examination of risks and benefits of pharmacotherapy during pregnancy and fetal and psychosocial risks related to untreated depression; examination of the safety of newer antidepressants to fetuses; examination of combination strategies; determination of the role of complementary medications and herbal remedies during pregnancy.
- Determination of the impact of maternal depression and elevated maternal cortisol on the developing fetal brain and later-life expression of the depressed phenotype in the child.
- Examination of interventions to target women for brief psychotherapeutic intervention strategies during periods of stress and vulnerability to relapse to reduce recurrence risk, including messages regarding sleep hygiene, avoidance of alcohol, and exercise (e.g., studies have found that monthly maintenance with interpersonal psychotherapy for depression for patients who have been successfully treated on an acute basis can be highly effective for women with recurrent depression [Frank et al. 2000]); conduct of studies on the efficacy of interpersonal psychotherapy and other psychotherapies with demonstrated efficacy for depression (e.g., CBT) as maintenance treatments.
- Development of outreach programs to target women at risk who may not have access to treatment; identification of women who need help through public health agencies, schools, places of worship, and other organizations; development of comanagement strategies with primary care providers so that psychiatrists are not simply waiting for referrals, while under-

detection in many primary care settings continues unabated; further study of team approaches incorporating case managers, social workers, home nurses, and support groups, such as the program at Medsplus Clinic, at the University of Michigan, in Ann Arbor. (This program provides women with transportation to the clinic and provides child care at the clinic. In addition, the program uses innovative techniques, such as interactive voice recognition, which allows women to use the telephone to access adjunctive treatment strategies, such as supportive therapy and CBT, and to participate in symptom monitoring in the privacy of their homes.)

- Development of better monitoring techniques, and incorporation of quality of life and global social functioning.

Conclusion

The devastating psychosocial consequences of undertreated depression in women include academic, developmental, and social decline in adolescence; marital and vocational disruption; loss of productivity and absenteeism in the workplace; disturbance of maternal-child bonding; and family discord. Suicide is a catastrophic result of depression. The untold human suffering makes depression among the most costly of disorders in both human and economic terms.

When properly treated, depression can be well controlled in many women, thus preventing much of this secondary morbidity. It is essential that we develop further strategies to minimize depressive recurrences in women to better address this common and treatable disorder.

References

Alpert JE, Fava M, Uebelacker LA, et al: Patterns of axis I comorbidity in early-onset versus late-onset major depressive disorder. Biol Psychiatry 46:202–211, 1999

Altemus AM, Kagan AE: Modulation of anxiety by reproductive hormones, in Gender Differences in Mood and Anxiety Disorders: From Bench to Bedside. Edited by Leibenluft E. Washington, DC, American Psychiatric Press, 1999, pp 53–90

Altshuler LL, Cohen L, Szuba MP, et al: Pharmacologic management of psychiatric illness during pregnancy: dilemmas and guidelines. Am J Psychiatry 153:592–606, 1996

Altshuler LL, Hendrick V, Cohen LS: Course of mood and anxiety disorders during pregnancy and the postpartum period. J Clin Psychiatry 59:9–33, 1998

American Psychiatric Association: Diagnostic and Statistical Manual of Mental Disorders, 3rd Edition. Washington, DC, American Psychiatric Association, 1980

American Psychiatric Association: Diagnostic and Statistical Manual of Mental Disorders, 4th Edition, Text Revision. Washington, DC, American Psychiatric Association, 2000

Amsterdam J, Garcia-Espana F, Fawcett J, et al: Fluoxetine efficacy in menopausal women with and without estrogen replacement. J Affect Disord 55:11–17, 1999

Angold A, Costello EJ, Erkanli A, et al: Pubertal changes in hormone levels and depression in girls. Psychol Med 29:1043–1053, 1999

Avis NE, Brambilla D, McKinlay SM, et al: A longitudinal analysis of the association between menopause and depression: results from the Massachusetts Women's Health Study. Ann Epidemiol 4:214–220, 1994

Baker A, Simpson S, Dawson D: Sleep disruption and mood changes associated with menopause. J Psychosom Res 43:359–369, 1996

Ballinger CB: Psychiatric aspects of the menopause. Br J Psychiatry 156:773–787, 1990

Berman AL, Jobes DA: Adolescent suicide assessment and intervention. Paper presented at the annual meeting of the American Psychiatric Association, Washington, DC, May 1991

Berndt ER, Koran LM, Finkelstein SN, et al: Lost human capital from early-onset chronic depression. Am J Psychiatry 157:940–947, 2000

Bifulco A, Brown GW, Moran P, et al: Predicting depression in women: the role of past and present vulnerability. Psychol Med 28:39–50, 1998

Blazer DG, Kessler RC, McGonagle KA, et al: The prevalence and distribution of major depression in a national community sample: the National Comorbidity Survey. Am J Psychiatry 151:979–986, 1994

Brady K: Depression treatment in menopausal women. Paper presented at the annual meeting of the American Psychiatric Association, Chicago, IL, May 2000

Briggs G, Freeman R, Yaffe S: Drugs in Pregnancy and Lactation, 5th Edition. Baltimore, MD, Williams & Wilkins, 1998, p xxii

Carranza-Lira S, Valentino-Figueroa ML: Estrogen therapy for depression in postmenopausal women. Int J Gynaecol Obstet 65:35–38, 1999

Castillo RJ: Culture and Mental Illness: A Client-Centered Approach. Pacific Grove, CA, Brooks/Cole, 1997, p 203

Chen IG, Roberts RE, Aday LA: Ethnicity and adolescent depression: the case of Chinese Americans. J Nerv Ment Dis 186:623–630, 1997

Choi WS, Patten CA, Gillin JC, et al: Cigarette smoking predicts development of depressive symptoms among US adolescents. Ann Behav Med 19:42–50, 1997

Cohen LS: Depression during pregnancy and postpartum. Presentation at Advances in Psychiatry, University of Michigan, Ann Arbor, November 2000

Cohen, LS, Rosenbaum G: Psychotropic drug use during pregnancy: weighing the risks. J Clin Psychiatry 59:18–28, 1998

Cohen LS, Friedman JM, Jefferson JW, et al: A reevaluation of risk of in utero exposure to lithium. JAMA 271:146–150, 1994

Cohen LS, Sichel DA, Robertson LM, et al: Postpartum prophylaxis for women with bipolar disorder. Am J Psychiatry 152:1641–1645, 1995

Cohen LS, Heller VL, Rosenbaum JF: Treatment guidelines for psychotropic drug use in pregnancy. Psychosomatics 30:25–33, 1998

Cooper PJ, Goodyer I: A community study of depression in adolescent girls. I: estimates of symptoms and syndrome prevalence. Br J Psychiatry 163:369–374, 1993

Coyne JC, Pepper C, Flynn HA: The significance of prior history of depression in two populations. J Consult Clin Psychol 67:76–81, 1999

Davies PT, Windle M: Gender-specific pathways between maternal depressive symptoms, family discord, and adolescent adjustment. Dev Psychol 33:657–668, 1997

Dolgan JI: Depression in children. Pediatr Ann 19:45–50, 1990

Egger HL, Angold A, Costello EJ: Headaches and psychopathology in children and adolescents. J Am Acad Child Adolesc Psychiatry 37:951–958, 1998

Emslie G, Rush A, Weinberg WA, et al: A double-blind, randomized, placebo-controlled trial of fluoxetine in children and adolescents with depression. Arch Gen Psychiatry 54:1031–1037, 1997

Ericson A, Kallen B, Wiholm B: Delivery outcome after the use of antidepressants in early pregnancy. Eur J Clin Pharmacol 55:503–508, 1999

Ernst C, Angst J: The Zurich Study, XII: sex differences in depression. Evidence from longitudinal epidemiological data. Eur Arch Psychiatry Clin Neurosci 241:222–230, 1992

Frank E, Thase ME: Natural history and preventative treatment of recurrent mood disorders. Annu Rev Med 50:453–468, 1999

Frank E, Carpenter LL, Kupfer DJ: Sex differences in recurrent depression: are there any that are significant? Am J Psychiatry 145:41–45, 1988

Frank E, Grochocinski VJ, Spanier CA, et al.: Interpersonal psychotherapy and antidepressant medication: evaluation of a sequential treatment strategy in women with recurrent major depression. J Clin Psychiatry 61:51–57, 2000

Geller B, Cooper TB, Graham DL, et al: Double-blind placebo-controlled study of nortriptyline in depressed adolescents using a "fixed plasma level" design. Psychopharmacol Bull 26:85–90, 1990

Ghaziuddin N, King CA, Hovey JD, et al: Medication noncompliance in adolescents with psychiatric disorders. Child Psychiatry Hum Dev 30:103–110, 1999

Ghaziuddin N, King CA, Naylor MW, et al: Anxiety contributes to suicidality in depressed adolescents. Depress Anxiety 11:134–138, 2000

Greden J, Tandon R: Long-term treatment for lifetime disorders? Arch Gen Psychiatry 52:197–200, 1995

Halbreich U, Rojansky N, Palter S, et al: Estrogen augments serotonergic activity in postmenopausal women. Biol Psychiatry 37:434–441, 1995

Harlow BL, Signorello LB: Factors associated with early menopause. Maturitas 35:3–9, 2000

Hay AG, Banckroft J, Johnstone EC: Affective symptoms in women attending a menopause clinic. Br J Psychiatry 164:513–516, 1994

Haynes P, Parry BL: Mood disorders and the reproductive cycle: affective disorders during the menopause and premenstrual dysphoric disorder. Psychopharmacol Bull 34:313–316, 1998

Hayward C, Gotlib IH, Schraedley PK: Ethnic differences in the association between pubertal status and symptoms of depression in adolescent girls. J Adolesc Health 25:143–149, 1999

Heim C, Nemeroff CB: The impact of early adverse experiences on brain systems involved in the pathophysiology of anxiety and affective disorders. Biol Psychiatry 46:1509–1522, 1999

Holte A: Menopause, mood and hormone replacement therapy: methodological issues. Maturitas 29:5–18, 1998

Hymas JS, Burke G, Davis PM, et al: Abdominal pain and irritable bowel syndrome in adolescents: a community-based study. J Pediatr 129:220–226, 1996

Jain J, Birmaher B, Garcia M, et al: Fluoxetine in children and adolescents with mood disorders: a chart review of efficacy and adverse effects. J Child Adolesc Pharmacol 2:267–275, 1992

Joffe H: Mood disorders in the perimenopause: the estrogen connection. Paper presented at the annual meeting of the American Psychiatric Association, Chicago, IL, May 2000

Joffe H, Cohen LS: Estrogen, serotonin and mood disturbance: where is the therapeutic bridge? Biol Psychiatry 44:798–811, 1998

Joffe H, Cohen LS, Hennen J, et al: The perimenopause is a period of risk for depressive symptoms in middle aged women. Paper presented at the annual meeting of the American Psychiatric Association, Washington DC, May 1999

Johnson BA, Roache JD, Javors MA, et al: Ondansetron for reduction of drinking among biologically predisposed alcoholic patients: a randomized controlled trial. JAMA 284:963–971, 2000

Jones KL, Lacro RV, Johnson KA, et al: Pattern of malformations in the children of women treated with carbamazepine during pregnancy. N Engl J Med 320:1661–1666, 1989

Kaminski KM, Naylor MW, King CA, et al: Reactive mood and atypical depression in psychiatrically hospitalized depressed adolescents. Depression 3:176–181, 1995

Kashani JH, Sherman DD: Childhood depression: epidemiology, etiological models, and treatment implications. Integrative Psychiatry 6:1–8, 1988

Kaufert PA, Gilbert P, Tate R: The Manitoba Project: a re-examination of the link between menopause and depression. Maturitas 14:143–155, 1992

Kessler RC, McGonagle KA, Swartz M, et al: Sex and depression in the National Comorbidity Survey, II: cohort effects. J Affect Disord 30:15–26, 1994a

Kessler RC, McGonagle KA, Zhao S, et al: Lifetime and 12-month prevalence of DSM-III-R psychiatric disorders in the United States: results from the National Comorbidity Survey. Arch Gen Psychiatry 51:8–19, 1994b

Klein DN, Schatzberg AF, McCullough JP, et al: Age of onset in chronic major depression: relation to demographic and clinical variables, family history, and treatment response. J Affect Disord 55:149–157, 1999

Kornstein SG: Gender differences in depression: implications for treatment. J Clin Psychiatry 58 (suppl 15):12–18, 1997

Kronenberg F: Hot flashes: phenomenology, quality of life, and search for treatment options. Exp Gerontol 29:319–336, 1994

Kulin NA, Pastuszak A, Sage SR, et al: Pregnancy outcome following maternal use of the new selective serotonin reuptake inhibitors: a prospective controlled multicenter study. JAMA 279:609–610, 1998

Kumar R, Robson MK: A prospective study of emotional disorders in childbearing women. Br J Psychiatry 144:35–47, 1984

Kurki T, Hileesmaa V, Raitasalo R, et al: Depression and anxiety in early pregnancy and risk for preeclampsia. Obstet Gynecol 95:487–490, 2000

Lammer EJ, Sever LE, Oakley GP Jr: Teratogen update: valproic acid. Teratology 35:465–473, 1987

Lehtinen V, Joukamaa M: Epidemiology of depression: prevalence, risk factors and treatment situation. Acta Psychiatr Scand Suppl 377:7–10, 1994

Lewinson PM, Zeiss AM, Duncan EM: Probability of relapse after recovery from an episode of depression. J Abnorm Psychol 98:107–116, 1989

Lindhout D, Meinardi H, Meijer JW, et al: Antiepileptic drugs and teratogenesis in two consecutive cohorts: changes in prescription policy paralleled by changes in pattern of malformations. Neurology 43:94–110, 1992

Marcus SM, Flynn HA, Barry KL, et al: Depression in pregnancy and postpartum: a review of critical issues. Postgraduate Obstetrics and Gynecology 20(13):1–8, 2000

Miller LJ: Clinical strategies for the use of psychotropic drugs during pregnancy. Psychiatric Medicine 9:275–298, 1991

Montgomery JC, Appleby L, Brincat M, et al: Effect of oestrogen and testosterone implants on psychological disorders in the climacteric. Lancet 1:297–299, 1987

Murray L: The impact of postnatal depression on infant development. J Child Psychol Psychiatry 33:543–561, 1992

Murray L, Hipwell A, Hooper R, et al: The cognitive development of 5-year-old children of postnatally depressed mothers. J Child Psychol Psychiatry 37:927–935, 1996

Myers JK, Weissman MM, Tischler GL, et al: Six-month prevalence of psychiatric disorders in three communities: 1980 to 1982. Arch Gen Psychiatry 41:959–967, 1984

National Center for Health Statistics: Advance report of final mortality statistics. Month Vital Stat Rep 39(4), 1990

Nicol-Smith L: Causality, menopause, and depression: a critical review of the literature. BMJ 313:1229–1232, 1996

Nolen-Hoeksema S: Epidemiology and theories of gender differences in unipolar depression, in Gender and Psychopathology. Edited by Seeman MV. Washington DC, American Psychiatric Press, 1995a, pp 63–87

Nolen-Hoeksema S: Gender differences in coping with depression across the lifespan. Depression 3:81–90, 1995b

Nulman I, Rovet J, Stewart DE, et al: Neurodevelopment of children exposed in utero to antidepressant drugs. N Engl J Med 336:258–262, 1997

O'Hara MW: Social support, life events, and depression during pregnancy and the puerperium. Arch Gen Psychiatry 43:569–573, 1986

Olsson G: Adolescent depression. Epidemiology, nosology, life stress and social network. Minireview based on a doctoral thesis. Ups J Med Sci 103:77–145, 1998

Omtzigt JGC, Los FJ, Grobbee DE, et al: The risk of spina bifida aperta after first-trimester exposure to valproate in a prenatal cohort. Neurology 42:119–125, 1992

Ostrov E, Offer D, Howard KI: Gender differences in adolescent symptomatology: a normative study. J Am Acad Child Adolesc Psychiatry 28:394–398, 1989

Pastuszak A, Shick-Boschetto B, Zuber C, et al: Pregnancy outcome following first-trimester exposure to fluoxetine. JAMA 269:2246–2248, 1993

Patton GC, Hibbert ME, Carlin J, et al: Menarche and the onset of depression and anxiety in Victoria, Australia. J Epidemiol Community Health 50:661–666, 1996

Pine DS, Cohen E, Cohen P, et al: Adolescent depressive symptoms as predictors of adult depression: moodiness or mood disorder? Am J Psychiatry 156:133–135, 1999

Prescott CA, Aggen SH, Kendler KS: Sex-specific genetic influences on the comorbidity of alcoholism and major depression in a population-based sample of US twins. Arch Gen Psychiatry 57:803–811, 2000

Rao U, Hammen C, Daley SE: Continuity of depression during the transition to adulthood: a 5-year longitudinal study of young women. J Am Acad Child Adolesc Psychiatry 38:908–915, 1999

Regier DA, Farmer ME, Rae DS, et al: One-month prevalence of mental disorders in the United States and sociodemographic characteristics. Acta Psychiatr Scand 88:35–47, 1994

Roberts RE, Roberts CR, Chen YR: Ethnocultural differences in prevalence of adolescent depression. Am J Community Psychol 25:95–110, 1997

Robinson J: Emergencies I, in Manual of Clinical Child Psychiatry. Edited by Robinson KS. Washington, DC, American Psychiatric Press, 1986, pp 185–211

Rubinow DR, Schmidt PJ, Roca CA: Estrogen-serotonin interactions: implications for affective regulation. Biol Psychiatry 44:839–850, 1998

Ryan ND, Puig-Antich J, Cooper T, et al.: Imipramine in adolescent major depression: plasma level and clinical response. Acta Psychiatr Scand 73:275–288, 1986

Schatzberg A: HPA axis interventions as treatment of depression. Paper presented at the annual meeting of the International Society for Psychoneuroendicrinology, San Francisco, CA, July 1998

Schmidt PJ, Rubinow DR: Menopause-related affective disorders: a justification for further study. Am J Psychiatry 148:844–852, 1991

Schmidt PJ, Roca CA, Rubinow DR: Clinical evaluation in studies of perimenopausal women: position paper. Psychopharmacol Bull 34: 309–311, 1998

Schwingl PJ, Hulka BS, Harlow SD: Risk factors for menopausal hot flashes. Obstet Gynecol 84:29–34, 1994

Sharp D, Hay DF, Pawlby S, et al: The impact of postnatal depression on boys' intellectual development. J Child Psychol Psychiatry 36:1315–1336, 1995

Sherwin BB: The impact of different doses of estrogen and progestin on mood and sexual behavior in postmenopausal women. J Clin Endocrinol Metab 72:336–343, 1991

Steer RA, Scholl TO, Hediger ML, et al: Self-reported depression and negative pregnancy outcomes. J Clin Epidemiol 45:1093–1099, 1992

Stowe ZN, Owens, MJ, Landry JC, et al: Sertraline and desmethylsertraline in human breastmilk and nursing infants. Am J Psychiatry 154: 1255–1260, 1997

Strober M, Freeman, R, Rigali J: The pharmacotherapy of depressive illness in adolescence: I. An open label trial of imipramine. Psychopharmacol Bull 26:80–84, 1990

Stuart S, O'Hara MW: Treatment of postpartum depression with interpersonal psychotherapy. Arch Gen Psychiatry 52:75–76, 1995

Tonkelaar ID, Oddens BJ: Determinants of long-term hormone replacement therapy and reasons for early discontinuation. Obstet Gynecol 95:507–512, 2000

Vamvakopoulos NS, Chrousos GP: Evidence of direct estrogenic regulation of human corticotropin-releasing hormone gene expression. J Clin Invest 92:1896–1902, 1993

Viguera AC, Nonacs R, Cohen LS, et al: Risk of recurrence of bipolar disorder in pregnant and nonpregnant women after discontinuing lithium maintenance. Am J Psychiatry 157:179–184, 2000

Weiss SR, Post RM: Kindling: separate vs. shared mechanisms in affective disorders and epilepsy. Neuropsychobiology 38:167–180, 1998

Weissman MM: Epidemiology of major depression in women: women and the controversies in hormonal replacement therapy. Paper presented at the annual meeting of the American Psychiatric Association, New York, May 1996

Weissman MM, Olfson M: Depression in women: implications for health care research. Science 269:799–801, 1995

Weissman MM, Leaf PJ, Tischler GL, et al: Affective disorders in five United States communities. Psychol Med 18:141–153, 1988

Weissman MM, Markowitz JC, Klerman GL: Comprehensive Guide to Interpersonal Psychotherapy. New York, Basic Books, 2000

Wheatley D: LI 160, an extract of St. John's wort, versus amitriptyline in mildly to moderately depressed outpatients—a controlled 6-week clinical trial. Pharmacopsychiatry 30 (suppl 2):77–80, 1997

Wilson N, Forfar JC, Goodman MJ: Atrial flutter in the newborn resulting from maternal lithium ingestion. Arch Dis Child 58:538–549, 1983

Wisner KL, Perel JM: Psychopharmacological treatment during pregnancy and lactation, in Psychopharmacology and Women: Sex, Gender and Hormones. Edited by Jensvold MF, Halbreich U, Hamilton JA. Washington DC, American Psychiatric Press, 1996, pp 191–224

Wisner KL, Perel JM, Findling RL: Antidepressant treatment during breast-feeding. Am J Psychiatry 153:1132–1137, 1996

Wisner KL, Gelenberg AL, Leonard H, et al: Pharmacologic treatment of depression during pregnancy. JAMA 282:1264–1269, 1999

Woody JN, London WL, Wilbanks GD: Lithium toxicity in a newborn. Pediatrics 47:94–96, 1971

Yoder MC, Belik J, Lannon RA, et al: Infants of mothers treated with lithium during pregnancy have an increased incidence of prematurity, macrostomia and perinatal mortality (abstract). Pediatr Res 18: 163A, 1984

Yonkers KA, Bradshaw KD: Hormone replacement and oral contraceptive therapy: do they induce or treat mood symptoms? in Gender Differences in Mood and Anxiety Disorders: From Bench to Bedside. Edited by Leibenluft E. Washington, DC, American Psychiatric Press, 1999, pp 91–35

Chapter 3

Chronic and Recurrent Depression

Pharmacotherapy and Psychotherapy Combinations

Robert Boland, M.D.
Martin B. Keller, M.D.

During the past two decades, substantial research data have demonstrated the need to view depression in longitudinal terms. Often viewed previously in episodic terms, depression, as we now understand, has a variety of possible courses and outcomes. Furthermore, we have increased our appreciation of the need to make treatment decisions with longitudinal assessments in mind.

Optimally, our goal is to prevent acute episodes of depression from developing into long-term disease. Though we have developed a number of effective treatments for major depression, much of what we know about these treatments involves the acute phase of treatment, and less is understood about continuation and maintenance treatment. The best treatment for chronic depression is remission, followed by sustained prophylactic treatment. The combination of different forms of treatment—specifically pharmacotherapy and psychotherapy—represents a new hope for optimizing treatment of depression.

Combination therapy has generally been thought to represent the best treatment for depression. This supposition, however, has largely been based on anecdotal and indirect data. Only recently have we begun to accumulate data to support the utility of combination therapy.

We begin this chapter by examining the varieties of long-term depression. We make the case that prospective long-term naturalistic studies and controlled treatment trials support the supposition that inadequate treatment of depression increases the risk of chronicity. We then review several studies of the treatment of chronic and recurrent depression. Finally, we examine some of the most pressing questions remaining about the treatment of long-term depression.

Importance of Adequate Treatment

Depression has a variety of long-term courses, and we continue to learn more about these. Most of what we know is derived from several naturalistic studies of the course of depression. One of the first was conducted by Angst (1986) in Zurich, in which 173 patients originally hospitalized for depression from 1959 to 1963 were followed up. Angst and colleagues (1973) found that although most patients recovered from their episodes of depression, a significant portion—about 13%— did not. This study followed up patients for as long as 21 years and concluded that a significant proportion of patients remained chronically depressed. In addition, they found the risk of recurrent depression to be surprisingly high, noting that three-quarters of patients eventually had at least one more episode of depression after recovering from the initial observed episode.

Similar results were observed in the clinical study associated with the Collaborative Depression Study (CDS) (Katz and Klerman 1979). CDS is the only other large, long-term, prospective naturalistic study of the course of depression. CDS followed up 555 patients who were experiencing a current episode of major depression. These patients were followed up every 6 months for 5 years and then annually for a minimum of 18 years. (Recent National Institute of Mental Health funding will extend the study to a minimum of 23 years.) CDS found that most patients recovered from their index episodes of depression within the first year of the study. However, for those who did not recover within the first year, the likelihood of recovery became greatly diminished. Thus, of the 33% of patients who did not recover within the first year, two-thirds did not recover by 2 years, about one-half did not recover by 5 years, and about one-fifth did not recover by 10 years. By 15 years, the rate of recovery leveled off, with about 6% of patients from the original sample still depressed.

CDS researchers had the advantage of prospectively observing subsequent episodes of depression (Keller and Boland 1998). Of patients in the study who experienced a second episode of depression, about 8% did not recover by 5 years. In an analysis that followed up individuals for a minimum of five prospective episodes, this probability of chronicity and time to recovery was similar for other subsequent prospectively observed episodes.

In essence, there is an additive risk of developing chronic depression with each subsequent episode. CDS indicated that for each episode, about 8% of patients would still be depressed within 5 years. The more episodes of depression a patient has, the more likely it will be for him or her to develop chronic depression, because the risk appears to increase arithmetically by another 8%. The importance, then, of preventing further episodes of depression is clear.

CDS also found the risk of recurrent depression to be high, indicating that the 2-year risk of recurrent depression was between 25% and 40%. These rates continued to increase over time. Patients had a 60% risk of recurrence after 5 years, 75% after 10 years, and 87% after 15 years. Thus, unlike the risk of chronicity, which seemed to reach a plateau for the sample, the risk of recurrence appeared to continually increase with time.

These data make clear the importance of adequately treating depression. Both the length and number of episodes of depression—the chronicity and recurrence rates—are risk factors for a long-term course.

Medication Treatment

Little data exist on the long-term treatment of depression, regardless of the intervention employed. What data do exist generally focus on the pharmacotherapy of depression. Six published studies have examined antidepressant treatment beyond the acute phase of treatment. Four studies used serotonin reuptake inhibitors: fluoxetine (Montgomery et al. 1988), paroxetine (Montgomery and Dunbar 1993), sertraline (Doogan and Caillard 1992), and citalopram (Montgomery et al. 1993). In the two other studies, Feiger et al. (1999) used nefazodone and Montgomery et al. (1998) used mirtazapine. Though the specific methodologies differed, in general, each study randomized patients to receive either a drug or placebo after an acute treatment phase. All were studies of continuation treatment (i.e., studies of the efficacy of these drugs in preventing relapse), and patients were examined for less than 1 year. In all studies, relapse rates were much higher among the placebo group (see Table 3–1). However, high rates of relapse, which increased with the length of the studies, were also found in most of the active treatment groups. In the longest studies, relapse rates were only marginally lower than rates found in the naturalistic studies, in which treatment was not controlled. Also of note is that in these studies, relapse tended to occur early—a high proportion of patients experienced a relapse within the first 2 to 4 months.

Few rigorous studies have been conducted on treatment beyond 1 year, but they are of particular importance because longer studies are required to examine the effectiveness of maintenance treatment. The goal of maintenance treatment is to prevent subsequent episodes of depression. Maintenance treatment is concerned with the prevention of *recurrence*, whereas acute treatment focuses on remission, and continuation treatment focuses on the prevention of relapse.

In a maintenance study, Prien and Kupfer (1986) examined patients successfully treated for acute depression during a 2-year period. Of the 150 patients beginning maintenance treatment, only 36% were successfully treated (i.e., they did not have a recurrence of depression during the 2-year maintenance period). The lowest rate of recurrence was in the patients receiving imipramine, alone or in combination with lithium. Even these patients, however, had a high rate of recurrence (47%). The maintenance doses used in that era were often less than therapeutic, and this was probably a factor in the high rate of recurrence (Figure 3–1).

Only a few studies have specifically targeted the treatment of patients with chronic or recurrent depression. Kocsis et al. (1996) reported on 14 patients with chronic depression who were includ-

Table 3–1. Relapse rates among patients who received continuation treatment (drugs versus placebo) for depression

Drug	Weeks of treatment	Drug relapse rate (%)	Placebo relapse rate (%)	P
Citalopram (Montgomery et al. 1993)	24	11	31	< 0.05
Fluoxetine (Montgomery et al. 1988)	52	26	57	< 0.01
Mirtazapine (Montgomery et al. 1998)	~30	4	28	< 0.05
Nefazodone (Feiger et al. 1999)	36	17	33	< 0.05
Paroxetine (Montgomery and Dunbar 1993)	52	16	43	< 0.001
Sertraline (Doogan and Caillard 1992)	44	13	46	< 0.001

Source. Keller MB, Kocsis JH, Thase ME, et al.: "Maintenance Phase Efficacy of Sertraline for Chronic Depression: A Randomized Controlled Trial." *Journal of the American Medical Association* 280:1665–1672, 1998.

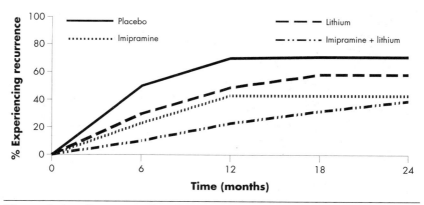

Figure 3–1. Outcome of maintenance treatment for patients with depression.

Note. Patients originally stabilized with lithium and imipramine were randomized to receive imipramine alone, lithium alone, both imipramine and lithium, or placebo. Imipramine was targeted to a dosage of 75 to 150 mg/day (average 135 mg/day), and lithium was targeted to a serum level of 0.6 to 0.9 mEq/L.

Source. Data from Prien RF, Kupfer DJ: "Continuation Drug Therapy for Major Depressive Episodes: How Long Should It Be Maintained?" *American Journal of Psychiatry* 143:18–23, 1986.

ed in a study of the use of desipramine for maintenance treatment of depression. Patients were initially treated for the acute episode of depression, and patients who experienced full or partial remission were entered in an open continuation phase of treatment, lasting 16 weeks. Of those completing this phase ($n = 60$), 3 fully remitted patients (5%) became partially remitted, 7 partially remitted patients (11%) became fully remitted, and 1 partially remitted patient (1%) had a relapse of depression. The responses to treatment in the majority of patients (83%) did not change.

Patients were then randomized into a maintenance phase of treatment, receiving either desipramine or placebo. These patients received maintenance treatment for up to 2 years. Patients receiving a placebo were four times more likely than the treatment group to have a recurrence of major depression.

Keller et al. (1995) studied a larger group of patients (631) with double depression or chronic major depression. These patients were treated with either sertraline or imipramine during the 12-week acute treatment phase; 60% of patients who completed this phase responded to treatment. However, the group treated with sertraline reported that the treatment was more tolerable, and the number of patients who discontinued treatment as a result of adverse events and the number of severe adverse events were significantly lower in this group. Patients who responded to treatment during the acute phase were entered into a 4-month, double-blind continuation phase of treatment. Of patients who fully responded to treatment during the acute phase, 71% and 73% who received sertraline and imipramine, respectively, continued to fully respond to treatment; 17% and 13% experienced a decline from full to partial response; and 12% and 15% lost treatment response during the continuation phase (Table 3–2). Of patients who partially responded to treatment during the acute phase and stayed on the same medication (double blinded), 51% and 45% who received sertraline and imipramine, respectively, experienced an increase from partial to full response; 34% and 27% maintained a partial response; and 15% and 29% lost treatment response during the continuation phase (Table 3–3). The 294 patients who responded were then randomized double blind to receive either sertraline or placebo during a 76-week maintenance treatment phase (Keller et al. 1998). As in the Kocsis et al. (1996) study, patients receiving a placebo were four times more likely to have a recurrence of depression. However, when analyzing rates of response during the different phases of treatment, it is clear that a sizable proportion of patients are not adequately treated by medication alone, and that patients who reach remission during the acute phase of treatment are more likely to maintain that remission and not lose their response during the subsequent 16 weeks of treatment with the same medication. This observation leads to the concept of combination therapy.

Combination Treatment

Cognitive Therapy and Pharmacotherapy for Depression Study

A study by Hollon et al. (1992) was one of first to use rigorous methodologies to compare psychotherapy and pharmacotherapy

Table 3–2. Outcome of continuation treatment among patients with depression who fully responded to acute-phase treatment

	Sertraline	Imipramine
n	140	88
Patients who discontinued treatment (%)	11	9
Patients whose response to treatment ended (%)	12	15
Patients whose response to treatment decreased from full to partial (%)	17	13
Patients who continued to fully respond to treatment (%)	71	73

Table 3–3. Outcome of continuation treatment among patients with depression who partially responded to acute-phase treatment

	Sertraline	Imipramine
n	99	59
Patients who discontinued treatment (%)	19	17
Patients whose response to treatment ended (%)	15	29
Patients who maintained partial response to treatment (%)	34	27
Patients whose response to treatment increased from partial to full (%)	51	45

Source.   Keller MB, Kocsis JH, Thase ME, et al.: "Maintenance Phase Efficacy of Sertraline for Chronic Depression: A Randomized Controlled Trial." *Journal of the American Medical Association* 280:1665–1672, 1998.

for the treatment of depression. The psychotherapy chosen for study was cognitive therapy.

Cognitive therapy is based on learning theory, in which it is believed that the maladaptive behaviors associated with depression are secondary to ingrained thoughts. These thoughts can lead to cognitive distortions, which are thought to be the basis of the "cognitive triad of depression": 1) negative self-view, 2) negative interpretation of past events, and 3) negative interpretation of the future. The goal of cognitive therapy is to recognize and question these distortions and, ultimately, correct distorted thoughts and behaviors. Similar to many behavioral therapies, cognitive therapy is active and requires a great deal of work outside the session in the form of homework. Treatment sessions are structured and can be taught with a manual. Thus, cognitive therapy lends itself well to investigation. Before the Hollon et al. (1992) study, researchers had accumulated extensive data showing the efficacy of cognitive therapy in treating depression, also making it an excellent choice for investigation.

In the study, 107 depressed patients were randomly assigned to receive cognitive therapy, imipramine, or a combination of the two. Patients eligible for this study had symptoms that met criteria for major depression as defined by Research Diagnostic Criteria (RDC), the Hamilton Rating Scale for Depression (HRSD; Hamilton 1960), and the Beck Depression Inventory (BDI; A. T. Beck et al. 1961). Patients with a history of most other major psychiatric disorders, including bipolar disorder or any psychotic disorder, were excluded.

Eighty percent of patients in this study were women, and 91% were Caucasian. The average age was 33 years, with a range of 18 to 62. Sixty-two percent of patients were employed outside the home; 13% were not. Almost half the patients had some college education, and patients were generally from lower-middle-class socioeconomic backgrounds. Marital status varied.

Sixty-four percent of patients had a history of recurrent depression, 37% had experienced three or more episodes of depression, and 24% had experienced double depression. The majority (66%) of patients had at least some suicidal ideation.

Patients were seen for an initial interview and at 6 weeks and 12 weeks after intake. Evaluation instruments included the HRSD, BDI, Raskin Depression Scale (Raskin et al. 1970), Global Assessment Scale (Endicott et al. 1976), and Minnesota Multiphasic Personality Inventory (Hathaway and McKinley 1951), which includes a depression subscale. Partial response was defined as a BDI score of 15 or less. Recovery was defined on the basis of improvement in these measures—particularly an HRSD score of 6 or greater and a BDI score of 9 or higher.

There was high attrition in this study: 55% of the patients who enrolled failed to initiate treatment, and 35% did not complete treatment. The rates of attrition did not differ by treatment modality.

Response rates during the acute treatment phase were 75% using the HRSD and 69% using the BDI, for patients who completed this phase of the study. Rates were lower if all patients enrolled were included—52% using the HRSD and 48% using the BDI.

Of patients who completed the acute treatment phase, those who at least partially responded to acute treatment were entered into a 2-year follow-up phase (Evans et al. 1992). Half the patients who took imipramine continued to take imipramine, and all other patients received placebo only. Evaluations during the follow-up phase consisted of monthly mailed questionnaires and 6-month in-person evaluations by a blinded evaluator. Assessments consisted of the HRSD and BDI and questions about relapse and participation in any treatment. Relapse during the follow-up phase was defined as two consecutive BDI scores of 16 or more, separated by at least 1 week.

Of the 64 patients who completed the acute treatment phase of the study, 50 were eligible for the follow-up phase. Of the 44 patients who participated in the follow-up phase, 38 either completed the study or experienced a relapse during it. The investigators found that 27% of patients experienced relapse during the 2 years of follow-up, based on the planned criteria. If the more liberal criterion of at least one elevated BDI score during the follow-up phase were used, 48% of the patients would have been judged to have relapsed.

The highest rate of relapse was in patients initially treated with imipramine and then randomized to the nonmedication group: 50% of these patients experienced relapse. Thirty-two percent of patients who continued to take imipramine, 21% of those who were treated with cognitive therapy, and 15% of those who received combination therapy experienced a relapse during the study.

The difference between the two cognitive therapy groups (i.e., the group treated with imipramine and the group treated without it) was not significant. However, when these two groups were pooled, it was found that they had less than half the relapse rate of those who had received medication and no continuation therapy.

This finding suggests that cognitive therapy confers a benefit, perhaps for years after it is discontinued. This differs from medication, for which benefits did not appear to be sustained once it was discontinued. In fact, there was an apparent detrimental effect to discontinuing medication, because the highest rate of relapse was seen in those who had been on medication and then discontinued the medication.

Pittsburgh Maintenance Therapies in Recurrent Depression

Pittsburgh Maintenance Therapies in Recurrent Depression (Frank et al. 1990) is a landmark study designed to investigate the role of treatment in preventing recurrent depression. According to the investigators, individuals were defined as having recurrent depression if 1) they were currently experiencing a third or higher episode of major depression, 2) the immediately preceding episode did not last longer than 2½ years before the onset of the current episode, and 3) a minimum of 10 weeks of remission occurred between the previous and index episodes. The latter criterion was meant to exclude patients with double depression. Patients underwent a 2-week drug-free "washout" period, after which they received combination therapy consisting of imipramine and interpersonal psychotherapy (IPT), which was continued until they showed a remission from the acute depressive episode.

IPT was chosen for the psychotherapy because it was developed specifically for the treatment of depression and a good deal of data support its use. Also, similar to cognitive therapy, IPT is structured and active. However, instead of focusing on thoughts and distortions, IPT focuses on improving a patient's relationships with others.

After remission, patients continued to receive combined treatment for 17 weeks, during which their remission had to remain stable. After this period, the patients who remained in remission were randomized into one of five maintenance treatments: 1) imipramine alone, 2) IPT alone, 3) IPT and imipramine, 4) IPT and placebo, or 5) placebo alone. This maintenance treatment was continued for 3 years. Of the 128 patients entering this phase of the study, 106 completed the protocol. During the maintenance phase, IPT sessions were done monthly, and the mean imipramine dosage during that period was 208 mg/day.

The group completing the 3-year maintenance phase had a mean survival time of 75.7 weeks, with a large variance in all treatment groups. The mean survival time, in order of survival, for each treatment group was 1) IPT and imipramine (131 weeks); 2) imipramine alone (124 weeks); 3) IPT alone (82 weeks); 4) IPT and placebo (74 weeks); and 5) placebo alone (45 weeks). These survival curves are illustrated in Figure 3–2. The patients taking imipramine had the highest chance for remaining well, and adding monthly IPT sessions did not confer an additional benefit.

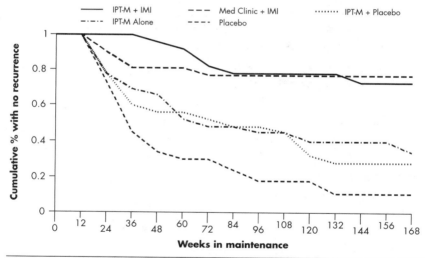

Figure 3–2. Mean survival time of patients who received full-dose maintenance treatment for depression.

Note. Average maintenance dosage of imipramine was 208 mg/day (50–350 mg/day). IPT-M = maintenance interpersonal psychotherapy; IMI = imipramine; Med Clinic = nonpsychotherapy visits for medication check.

Source. Data from Frank E, Kupfer DJ, Perel JM, et al.: "Three-Year Outcomes for Maintenance Therapies in Recurrent Depression." *Archives of General Psychiatry* 47:1093–1099, 1990.

Following the maintenance period, the study was extended for another 2 years (Kupfer et al. 1992). Participants were drawn from the patients who completed the 3 years of maintenance in either of the two medication groups (with or without IPT). These patients were continued in the same psychotherapy condition they had before (with or without IPT) and were randomized to receive imipramine or placebo. Of the 28 patients eligible for this phase of the study, 20 entered. Eleven of the patients received imipramine, and 6 of these also received IPT. Seven of the placebo patients also received IPT. Of the 20 patients beginning the study, 7 had a recurrence of depression. Only 1 patient in the medication group had a recurrence (and the serum imipramine level suggested noncompliance), whereas 6 out of 9 of the placebo patients experienced a relapse during the 2 years. The mean survival time in the active treatment group was about 100 weeks, versus 54 weeks in the placebo group. These data suggest that effective maintenance treatment is possible and that there are potential advantages to combination therapies, although the low frequency of IPT in the study (monthly) did not maximize the likelihood that IPT would have a beneficial effect.

Geriatric Depression Study

The Geriatric Depression Study was similar in design to Pittsburgh Maintenance Therapies in Recurrent Depression, except that it focused on elderly patients (Reynolds et al. 1999). Another difference was in the use of nortriptyline instead of imipramine, chosen because of its better side-effect profile in elderly patients. Patients older than 59 years with recurrent depression were recruited for the study; 187 patients were entered into the study. Of these, 107 were fully recovered after acute treatment with nortriptyline and IPT. These patients were randomly assigned to one of four maintenance therapy interventions: 1) medication alone, 2) medication and IPT, 3) IPT and placebo, or 4) placebo alone. The psychotherapy was administered once a week. Nortriptyline blood levels were kept between 80 and 120 ng/mL.

Maintenance treatment was continued for 3 years. Recurrence rates during this period were as follows: combined treatment, 20%; medication alone, 43%; IPT plus placebo, 64%; and placebo alone, 90%. Thus, another study suggests the superiority of combination therapy.

Treatment of Chronic Depression Study

Some of the strongest data justifying the use of combination therapy for long-term treatment of depression come from a multicenter trial conducted by Keller et al. (2000). In this study, 681 patients from 12 different sites were randomly assigned to receive acute therapy for depression. The treatments consisted of nefazodone and psychotherapy, alone and in combination. The psychotherapy was the cognitive behavioral–analysis system of psychotherapy developed by McCullough (1995), a structured form of cognitive behavioral therapy that includes elements of IPT.

In the study, the acute treatment phase continued for 12 weeks. Patients who did not respond to treatment were crossed over to another 12 weeks of treatment with an alternative therapy. (Patients who did not respond to combination therapy were discontinued from the study.)

Patients who responded to treatment during the acute phase then received 16 weeks of continuation treatment or the same therapy used in the acute phase. Patients who responded to treatment and experienced remission during the continuation phase then entered a 1-year maintenance study, which was a double-blind randomization to active treatment or placebo. Response was defined as a decrease of at least 50% in HRSD score from baseline to weeks 10 and 12, with a total score of 15 or lower at weeks 10 and 12, but a total score of higher than 8 at weeks 10, 12, or both. Remission was defined as an HRSD score of no more than 8 at both weeks 10 and 12 for those completing the acute phase protocol (or at the time of withdrawal for those who did not).

In the acute phase, the combination therapy group had the highest attainment of total remission—85% compared with 55% in the group that received medication only and 52% in the group that received psychotherapy only. The results of an intention-to-treat analysis were just as striking: 73% of patients in the combination therapy group showed a total response, compared with 48% for the medication-only group and 47% for the psychotherapy-

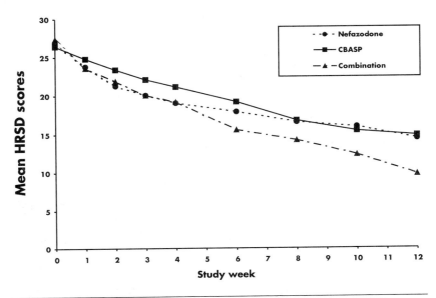

Figure 3–3. Mean Hamilton Rating Scale for Depression (HRSD) scores of patients treated with nefazodone, cognitive-behavioral therapy, or both. *Note.* Mean dosage of nefazodone for patients completing the study was 520 mg/day in the nefazodone group and 479 mg/day in the combined treatment group. CBASP = cognitive behavioral–analysis system of psychotherapy. *Source.* Reprinted with permission from Keller MB, McCullough JP, Klein DN, et al.: "A Comparison of Nefazodone, the Cognitive Behavioral–Analysis System of Psychotherapy, and Their Combination for the Treatment of Chronic Depression." *New England Journal of Medicine* 342:1462–1470, 2000. Copyright © 2000 Massachusetts Medical Society. All rights reserved.

only group (Figure 3–3). These combination therapy response rates are the highest reported to date in a large-scale controlled trial for major depression.

In an examination of differential response, the time course was important. Earlier response was seen in the medication-only group. The positive effects of psychotherapy alone or in combination with pharmacotherapy became apparent only after 4 weeks of treatment. Thus, the effects did not appear to be merely additive. This concept may be important in explaining the apparent benefits of combination therapy.

This study lends great support for using both medication and psychotherapy in the treatment of chronically depressed patients and suggests that the two treatments should be begun simultaneously. Also of note is the intensive nature of the psychotherapy—the therapy was given 16 to 20 times over 12 weeks, with up to two sessions per week during the first 6 weeks.

Data from the continuation, crossover, and maintenance phases should soon be available and should answer several critical hypotheses about combination therapy in the longer term.

Current Issues, Unanswered Questions

Despite having limitations, the aforementioned studies represent major advances in our understanding of the treatment of depression. Although many questions exist regarding the best management for patients with chronic or recurrent depression, these studies begin to answer some of these questions.

Perhaps the most important question is whether combination therapy is preferable to either medication treatment or psychotherapy alone for patients with long-term depressive disorders. In the studies discussed here, combination therapy was clearly preferable to psychotherapy alone. However, only partially answered until recently was the question of whether adding psychotherapy to a medication regimen is preferable to medication alone. Most studies showed some benefit from combination therapy, but some of the earlier studies demonstrated only modest improvements from the addition of psychotherapy to medication treatment. Looking at these data, one might wonder from a cost-benefit perspective whether the expense and time of adding psychotherapy are justified. It is for this reason that the study by Keller et al. (2000) is important. This study showed, by far, the most robust benefit from combination therapy. Combination treatment increased response rates from approximately 50% to approximately 85%. It is not clear why the differences observed in this study are so much more striking than those observed in previous studies, though it may relate to the high intensity of psychotherapy given and to progressive improvements in the techniques of specific cognitive therapies used and the training of those administering the treatments. If these figures are confirmed by other studies, the benefits of combination therapy over monotherapy will shift the burden of proof even further: rather than justifying combination therapy, clinicians will have to justify why a patient is not receiving combination therapy.

A second question is whether the additional benefits of combination therapy are merely additive or whether they have differential/complementary effects. Are certain symptoms more amenable to one type of therapy than to another? Certainly, in clinical practice, treatment choices are often the result of these assumptions. The study by Reynolds et al. (1999) employed IPT with the assumption that it would be a good complement to medication, because many elderly people are thought to have depressive symptoms as a result of interpersonal losses. However, most of the studies do not report on whether certain symptoms differentially improve with one type of treatment or another. Indirect evidence for differential effect is seen in the Keller et al. (2000) study, in that the time to recovery differed in the psychotherapy groups and the pharmacotherapy groups. This suggests a possible independent effect for the two treatments. Certainly, the possibility of independent effects should be the subject of future research.

A study by Ravindran et al. (1999) found that patients with dysthymia who were treated with combination therapy were more likely to improve in certain specific coping strategies. Though patients treated with monotherapy (sertraline or cognitive-behavioral therapy alone) improved overall in depression ratings, their coping styles did not change in a manner similar to the combination therapy group. Thus, it is possible that combination therapy also offers specific advantages over monotherapy in its ability to attack certain symptoms or behaviors, though this needs to be investigated further.

In addition to varying effects on specific symptoms, the use of different but complementary treatments may offer other benefits. For example, in the Cognitive Therapy and Pharmacotherapy for Depression Study described previously (Hollon et al. 1992), patients who received cognitive therapy were less likely to have a relapse later, even after their treatment was discontinued, than those treated solely with medication after their treatment was discontinued. This finding validates the presumption that cognitive therapy is a type of learning. Thus, it can catalyze long-lasting changes in thoughts and coping strategies. Although there are mechanisms that might explain long-term positive changes that follow maintenance medication after it is discontinued (e.g., persistent alterations in gene expression), available data do not support that explanation. In fact, in this study, the medication-only group had the highest rate of relapse after discontinuation of treatment, confirming the growing clinical suggestion that for many patients there is a strong detrimental effect associated with stopping antidepressant treatment. It is reasonable to hypothesize that, in the subgroup of patients who strenuously insist on avoiding long-term medication treatment, psychotherapy may be a crucial ingredient in lowering their risk for relapse.

The possibility of other complementary effects from combination therapy should be considered. For example, there are reasons to believe that psychotherapy can enhance treatment adherence (see J. S. Beck 2001).

Other questions about combination therapy also beg for answers, and they are already being debated among clinicians. One question is whether it is preferable or detrimental to split the psychotherapy and psychopharmacology among different treatment providers. Some of the possible pitfalls and benefits of such a split are discussed elsewhere (see Riba and Balon 2001). The studies discussed here cannot answer the question because there were no "head-to-head" comparisons, but it is notable that in the design of all studies, the therapies were split (i.e., administered by different clinicians).

Another important question pertains to the economic analyses for combination therapy. The World Health Organization reports that depression is the most important cause of disability in developed countries (Murray and Lopez 1996). Given the economic burden of depression and emerging data, one can make a strong argument for adding psychotherapy to medication treatment alone, for economic reasons as well as outcome reasons, particularly if the robust results reported by Keller et al. (2000) are replicated by others.

Conclusion

During the 1990s, we learned a great deal about the treatment of chronic and recurrent depression. There is, however, still much to be done, but evidence is emerging that supports the use of combined psychopharmacology and psychotherapy:

- Combination therapy appears to be more effective than either medication treatment or psychotherapy alone for the treatment of chronic and recurrent major depression.
- It appears that psychotherapy must be of sufficient intensity and duration to truly add to the pharmacology effect. This may mean that sessions must be conducted at a higher frequency than is currently practiced.
- Several patient populations may particularly benefit from combination therapy: 1) patients with chronic depression (Keller et al. 2000), 2) "old-old" patients with depression (Reynolds et al. 1999), and 3) patients with recurrent depression who insist on discontinuing medication (these patients should be strongly advised to undergo psychotherapy before medication is discontinued).
- Strong evidence supports the use of cognitive-behavioral therapy and IPT as monotherapies for depression. Nevertheless, the type of psychotherapy that is best suited for combination therapy needs to be determined, because studies have not compared multiple psychotherapies.
- Whether there is a medication that is best suited for combination therapy is not clear. As with monotherapy, all antidepressants are likely to be efficacious and effective, and medication decisions will likely focus on the traditional issues of safety, adherence, acceptable side-effect profiles, pharmacokinetics, and cost. Data exist on only a few medications used in combination therapy, notably the tricyclic antidepressant imipramine and the newer agent nefazodone. Of those two agents, nefazodone is likely to have the preferable tolerability for most patients.

Further study and longer follow-ups are essential. Replication of the study by Keller et al. (2000) may promote an important change in the way maintenance antidepressant treatment is practiced. Certainly, for many clinicians, these findings will merely confirm what has long been suspected. For others, it will force them to tackle some biases. The health care industry has been biased against the use of psychotherapy, pointing to the lack of data and the cost to justify its bias. Furthermore, many insurance companies and health maintenance organizations have treated all psychotherapies (and psychotherapists) equally. These biases must be reconsidered.

The psychotherapies used in the studies discussed in this chapter are very explicit in their techniques and goals, are targeted specifically for depression, and require special training. With data such as those presented here, the burden of proof may shift dramatically, and in the future, clinicians may have to justify their reasons for not using combination therapy and, specifically, certain types of therapy for specific conditions.

References

Angst J: The course of major depression, atypical bipolar disorder, and bipolar disorder, in New Results in Depression Research. Edited by Hippius H. Berlin/Heidelberg, Springer-Verlag, 1986, pp 26–35

Angst J, Baastrup P, Grof P, et al: The course of monopolar depression and bipolar psychoses. Psychiatria, Neurologia, Neurochirurgia 76: 489–500, 1973

Beck AT, Ward CH, Mendelsohn M, et al: An inventory for measuring depression. Arch Gen Psychiatry 4:561–571, 1961

Beck JS: A cognitive therapy approach to medication compliance, in Integrated Treatment of Psychiatric Disorders (Review of Psychiatry Series, Volume 20, Number 2; Oldham JM and Riba MB, series editors). Edited by Kay J. Washington, DC, American Psychiatric Publishing, 2001

Doogan DP, Caillard V: Sertraline in the prevention of depression. Br J Psychiatry 160:217–222, 1992

Endicott J, Spitzer RL, Fleiss JL, et al: The global assessment scale: a procedure for measuring overall severity of psychiatric disturbance. Arch Gen Psychiatry 33:766–771, 1976

Evans MD, Hollon SD, DeRubeis RJ, et al: Differential relapse following cognitive therapy and pharmacotherapy for depression. Arch Gen Psychiatry 49:802–808, 1992

Feiger AD, Bielski RJ, Bremner J, et al: Double-blind placebo-substitution study of nefazodone in the prevention of relapse during continuation treatment of outpatients with major depression. Clin Psychopharmacol 14:19–28, 1999

Frank E, Kupfer DJ, Perel JM, et al: Three-year outcomes for maintenance therapies in recurrent depression. Arch Gen Psychiatry 47:1093–1099, 1990

Hamilton MA: A rating scale for depression. J Neurol Neurosurg Psychiatry 23:56–62, 1960

Hathaway SR, McKinley JC: The Minnesota Multiphasic Personality Inventory Manual. New York, Psychological Corp, 1951

Hollon SD, DeRubeis RJ, Evans MD, et al: Cognitive therapy and pharmacotherapy for depression: singly and in combination. Arch Gen Psychiatry 49:774–781, 1992

Katz M, Klerman GL: Introduction: overview of the clinical studies program. Am J Psychiatry 136:49–51, 1979

Keller MB, Boland RJ: Implications of failing to achieve successful long-term maintenance treatment of recurrent unipolar major depression. Biol Psychiatry 44:348–360, 1998

Keller MB, Harrison W, Fawcett JA, et al: Treatment of chronic depression with sertraline or imipramine: preliminary blinded response rates and high rates of undertreatment in the community. Psychopharmacol Bull 31:205–212, 1995

Keller MB, Kocsis JH, Thase ME, et al: Maintenance phase efficacy of sertraline for chronic depression: a randomized controlled trial. JAMA 280:1665–1672, 1998

Keller MB, McCullough JP, Klein DN, et al: A comparison of nefazodone, the cognitive behavioral–analysis system of psychotherapy, and their combination for the treatment of chronic depression. N Engl J Med 342:1462–1470, 2000

Kocsis JH, Friedman RA, Markowitz JC, et al: Maintenance therapy for chronic depression: a controlled clinical trial of desipramine. Arch Gen Psychiatry 53:769–774, 1996

Kupfer DJ, Frank E, Perel JM, et al: Five-year outcome for maintenance therapies in recurrent depression. Arch Gen Psychiatry 49:769–773, 1992

McCullough JP: Therapist Manual for Cognitive Behavioral Analysis System of Psychotherapy. Richmond, VA, Virginia Commonwealth University, 1995

Montgomery SA, Dunbar G: Paroxetine is better than placebo in relapse prevention and the prophylaxis of recurrent depression. Int Clin Psychopharmacol 8:189–195, 1993

Montgomery SA, Dunfour H, Brion S, et al: The prophylactic efficacy of fluoxetine in unipolar depression. Br J Psychiatry 153 (suppl 3):69–76, 1988

Montgomery SA, Rasmussen JG, Tanghoj P: A 24-week study of 20 mg citalopram, 40 mg citalopram, and placebo in the prevention of relapse of major depression. Int Clin Psychopharmacol 8:181–188, 1993

Montgomery SA, Reimitz PE, Zivkov M: Mirtazapine versus amitriptyline in the long-term treatment of depression: a double-blind placebo-controlled study. Int Clinical Psychopharmacol 13:63–73, 1998

Murray CJL, Lopez AD: Global Burden of Disease and Injury Series, Vol l: The Global Burden of Disease: A Comprehensive Assessment of Mortality and Disability from Diseases, Injuries and Risk Factors in 1990 and Projected to 2020. Boston, MA, Harvard University Press, 1996

Prien RF, Kupfer DJ: Continuation drug therapy for major depressive episodes: how long should it be maintained? Am J Psychiatry 143:18–23, 1986

Raskin A, Schulterbrandt JG, Reating N, et al: Differential response to chlorpromazine, imipramine and placebo. Arch Gen Psychiatry 23:164–173, 1970

Ravindran AV, Anisman H, Merali Z, et al: Treatment of primary dysthymia with group cognitive therapy and pharmacotherapy: clinical symptoms and functional impairments. Am J Psychiatry 156:1608–1617, 1999

Reynolds CF III, Frank E, Perel JM, et al: Nortriptyline and interpersonal psychotherapy as maintenance therapies for recurrent major depression: a randomized controlled trial in patients older than 59 years. JAMA 281:39–45, 1999

Riba MB, Balon R: The challenges of split treatment, in Integrated Treatment of Psychiatric Disorders (Review of Psychiatry series, Vol 20, No 2; Oldham JM and Riba MB, series editors). Edited by Kay J. Washington, DC, American Psychiatric Publishing, 2001

Chapter 4

Prevention of Recurrences in Patients With Bipolar Disorder

The Best of the Old and the New

Charles L. Bowden, M.D.
Cheryl L. Gonzales, M.D.

The cornerstone of maintenance treatment for patients with bipolar disorder is effectively using a recently expanded group of drugs that, alone or in combination, provide a good chance of prophylaxis against new episodes; maintaining subthreshold symptomatology at levels compatible with good function; and yielding tolerability that neither impairs function nor predisposes patients to nonadherence to the treatment regimen. The goals of maintaining remission and good function are eminently achievable, yet they are elusive, because of the inherent complexities of bipolar disorder.

Goals of Care for Patients With Bipolar Disorder

Importance of Illness-Focused Treatment

Maintenance treatment of bipolar disorder should be illness-focused, not episode-focused. Most patients with bipolar disorder have some minor symptoms between episodes, even during periods of sustained remission. Two lines of evidence recommend that clinicians pay attention to these between-episode manifestations of the disorder. First, subthreshold symptoms, but not relapse into new episodes, have been significantly associated with functional episode outcomes in bipolar disorder (Gitlin et al. 1995). Second, functional recovery has been delayed by several months following remission of a full episode (Horgan 1981; Tohen et al. 2000a).

An illness focus also helps the patient recognize milder symptoms that may serve as warning indicators of the need for change in the treatment regimen. Illness-focused care provides the best chance of good function and of keeping treatment costs low. The treatment costs of bipolar disorder are heavily driven by the costs of hospitalization and emergency room evaluation for full-episode relapses. A corollary is that treatment visits need to be regular and frequent, even for well-functioning patients. Our practice is to schedule 4 to 12 visits per year visits for patients who are doing well, unless unusual circumstances require otherwise. Illness-focused care also facilitates the following goals: family involvement, recognition of risk factors for relapse, and keeping the patient in treatment.

Family Involvement

We usually encourage family members to attend at least some appointments. However, there will be instances when this is counterproductive (e.g., unmarried adults may feel that ongoing family involvement interferes with their autonomy, or family involvement may contribute to intrusive, stressful interactions between the patient and a family member). Usually, however, advantages accrue. The family can learn about the illness along with the patient. Family members often become sensitive to highly characteristic, idiosyncratic early warning signs of relapse (e.g., an escalating interest in a field of endeavor, telling off-color jokes, or a change in dress). Although such symptoms may constitute an expression of illness in a particular patient, they often do not meet DSM-IV-TR criteria for the diagnosis of mania (American Psychiatric Association 2000) and thus might be overlooked.

Certain behaviors that are often not recognized by patients despite their best intentions are recognized by family. These include impulsive risk-taking, quick onset of irritability, and preoccupations that suggest self-referential thinking (e.g., intense attention to national news, with the belief that the events are in some way self-pertinent). Without family involvement, there is a substantial likelihood that some or all of these behaviors will go unrecognized by even an astute psychiatrist who sees his or her patient regularly. Illness-defining behaviors may go unrecognized if the patient does not demonstrate such behaviors during appointments, if the psychiatrist does not recognize that the behavior is untoward, or if the behavior does not occur infrequently or occurs only under certain circumstances. In addition, if the family has unrealistic expectations of the patient, these expectations can be made commensurate with treatment goals. Finally, the family can play a positive role in its actions with the patient between visits.

Recognition of Risk Factors for Relapse

Many risk factors for relapse are identifiable and, to a certain degree, under voluntary control. Risk factors for mania are similar to those for mixed states and hypomania. Therefore, although "mania" will be the term used in this chapter, all three of these states are implied.

Inadequate Sleep

Inadequate sleep, especially if sustained over several days, predisposes patients with bipolar disorder to hypomanic states (Goodwin and Jamison 1990). Some patients become aware of this and deliberately limit sleep to deal with depressive symptoms. Shift work; long work hours, particularly in training positions such as internships; and studying late at night can result in inadequate sleep. Police and health care personnel are especially vulnerable to these chronobiological shifts. Sleep difficulties during the last trimester of pregnancy and during the postpartum period may contribute to increased risk of mood episodes.

Drugs and Medical Disorders

Drugs and medical disorders that have been reported to cause mania in patients with bipolar disorder are listed in Table 4–1. The risk of mania from these varies. Although stimulants may destabilize mood, the number of such reports is small, and stim-

Table 4–1. Drugs and medical disorders that predispose to exacerbation of bipolar disorder

Drugs	Medical conditions
Alcohol	AIDS
Anabolic steroids	Brain trauma
Antidepressants	Brain tumors, other space occupying lesions
Corticosteroids	Cushing's syndrome
Hallucinogens	Encephalitis
Interferon	Multiple sclerosis
Isoniazid	
Sympathomimetic agents	

ulants have been reported to be effective in reducing mania (Garvey et al. 1987). Furthermore, concurrent use of stimulants and valproate or lithium by adolescents with mania and concurrent symptoms of attention-deficit/hyperactivity disorder indicate that benefits from the combination treatment may occur, rather than detrimental effects.

Increased Exposure to Light

Increased exposure to light may predispose a patient with bipolar disorder to mania. This is most associated with seasonal shifts in risk, with a strong counter-risk for depression in the autumn (Silverstone et al. 1995). Artificial light and air travel that extends the period of daylight may also contribute to mania risk. It is unclear whether the risk mechanism is simply disruption of sleep or whether the risk is mediated via serotonin, melatonin, or other circadian pacemaking abnormality that may be associated with the pathophysiology of bipolar disorder. Recent discovery of the "clock" gene, which in part controls circadian rhythmicity, presents an opportunity to develop model systems and drugs relevant to the pathophysiology and/or treatment of bipolar disorder. Attention to all these factors can be rewarding, in part because they are ones that patients can come to recognize and control, thereby reducing any sense of futility and increasing confidence about the future. For example, recognizing that some of the detrimental effects of substance abuse in general and alcoholism in particular comes from interference with sleep may aid in commitment to reduce drinking.

Excitement and Stressors

Excitement and stressors also predispose patients with bipolar disorder to mania. It is likely that autonomic activation and hypothalamic-pituitary-adrenocortical (HPA) system activation are mediating factors. Substantial data on hypercortisolism in mixed mania provide inferential evidence of such a link (Evans and Nemeroff 1983; Krishnan et al. 1983; Swann et al. 1990). Additionally, more recent studies on persisting system overactivity as a result of maternal deprivation in early life provide a possible mechanism by which some patients might be at higher risk for mania (Nemeroff 1998).

Keeping the Patient in Treatment

Bipolar disorder is a highly recurrent, lifelong disease. There is evidence that a greater number of lifetime episodes predisposes patients to a poor response to lithium, although not to divalproex sodium (Gelenberg et al. 1989; Swann et al. 1999). In a 1-year study of maintenance treatment with lithium or divalproex sodium, the total treatment costs for patients who took medication 3 months or more were less than one-third the costs for patients who stopped taking medication within the first 3 months (Hirschfeld et al. 1999). Almost all the increased costs were associated with higher relapse rates and subsequent need for hospitalization. The implications of these findings are underscored by a large study showing that the mean duration of continuous lithium use by patients with bipolar I disorder was 65 days, despite intentions to use lithium as prophylactic therapy (Johnson and McFarland 1996).

Using medications with good to excellent tolerability is among the most important steps a psychiatrist can take to keep the patient in treatment. The adverse effect profile and safety index of lithium are among the most difficult to overcome in all of medicine. However, even with lithium, many patients can achieve a balance of effective and adequately tolerated dosing. It is likely that the published low tolerability of lithium is worse than can often be achieved, because lithium was for many years the only available treatment for bipolar disorder. Therefore, psychiatrists tended to deal with adverse effects by encouraging patients to put up with them, and dealt with any worsening of the illness by increasing dosage. With a wider range of available treatments, psychiatrists should test lower doses of any mood-stabilizing drug when patients have even subjective, or cosmetic, distress. There is sufficient evidence that lithium and divalproex sodium require serum levels of 0.8 mEq/L and 45 µg/mL, respectively, for efficacy in treating bipolar I mania; however, data regarding maintenance dosing and efficacy are meager and inconsistent. What is clear is that adverse effects worsen in number and severity with higher doses (Bowden et al. 2000; Gelenberg et al. 1989; Vestergaard et al. 1998). Additionally, some patients do well with substantially lower levels of lithium or valproate and possibly other drugs. Therefore, in the face of any adverse effect to patients, we encourage a cautious test of lowering dosage, use of sustained-release formulations, and consideration of combining an effective but poorly tolerated drug with a complementary drug that might allow a lower dose of the former. If these strategies fail, we recommend discontinuation of the drug and the use of other agents.

It is important to attend assiduously to other factors that cause patients to drop out of treatment. Many patients with unequivocal bipolar disorder are highly opposed to acknowledging that they have the disorder. For some patients, it may be helpful to establish a therapeutic relationship through regular visits and to use medications that are helpful in treating at least a portion of the illness, while working with the patient to overcome his or her resistance to acknowledging the disorder. A common variant is the patient who acknowledges that he or she has had bipolar disorder, but views a relatively illness-free period as evidence of cure and as an indicator that further treatment is not needed. We are increasingly inclined to view such behavior not just as poor insight, which might lead to recrudescence of the illness, but as a primary symptom of the illness that warrants intervention. For some patients, signed agreements allowing the psychiatrist to intervene in an unconventional way if the patient becomes manic or depressed can be helpful. Missed appointments need to be promptly followed up and the family and significant others must be involved.

Therapeutic Relationships

All medical care is built around therapeutic relationships. Such relationships are more critical and complex when the disease is lifelong, multidimensional, associated with inherited factors, and worsened or improved by common environmental factors. Bipolar disorder has all these characteristics. Little systematic study of psychosocial factors or specific psychotherapy in bipolar disorder has been published. Counseling has resulted in higher rates of treatment continuation, a primary treatment objective in our view (Miklowitz and Goldstein 1990). Kay Redfield Jamison, a psychologist who has written extensively and movingly of her experience with bipolar disorder, has emphasized the value of a strong therapeutic relationship and often psychotherapy (Jamison 1995).

There are many benefits that can be derived from the therapeutic relationship. The patient gains information about a strange and complex disorder, much of which is learned over time, in the context of the patient's current circumstances, and gradually comes to identify himself or herself as having an illness. Two key facets of the therapeutic relationship are the structure provided by scheduled visits and the systematic attention given to symptoms and illness factors. The therapeutic relationship provides the patient with a knowledgeable, caring person to contact and helps the patient keep appointments, continue to take medication, and apply a relatively structured routine to his or her daily life.

Frank incorporated many of these notions into a semistructured social rhythm psychotherapy (Frank et al. 1994). No evidence of benefits from this psychotherapy has been published; however, two more recent studies suggest that the benefits of an effective therapeutic relationship occur for bipolar patients with mania, rather than for those with depression. In the first study (Bowden et al. 2000), outcomes of a 1-year maintenance study comparing patients randomized to blinded treatment with divalproex sodium, lithium, or placebo were more positive for the placebo group than had been predicted. In contrast to a predicted rate of mania relapse with placebo of 55%, only 19% developed mania. Other factors contributed to these results. Patients taking lithium were slowly tapered off at the time of randomization to avoid abrupt discontinuation-induced relapses. (Abrupt discontinuation of lithium at the time of randomization increased relapse rates in earlier studies of lithium in prophylactic treatment.) Also, more patients with somewhat milder forms of bipolar disorder may have been enrolled. However, we believe it is likely that the effective therapeutic relationships, which are characteristic of most good-quality drug treatment studies, contributed to good outcomes. All patients received 1) effective supportive psychotherapy, inculcating all the principles discussed in this chapter, 2) education about the disorder and its treatment, and 3) systematic attention to all aspects of the illness from well-qualified staff. In addition, patients made frequent treatment visits (once a week to every 4 weeks) and were promptly contacted if they missed a visit. Of interest, the drug-placebo differences in the study were modest regarding mania relapse but significantly favored divalproex sodium over placebo on depressive relapse.

A second recent study (Calabrese et al. 2000) provides further inferential evidence that bipolar patients experiencing mania obtain much benefit from a structured therapeutic relationship. Patients with rapid-cycling bipolar disorder were treated with lamotrigine alone or placebo for 12 weeks in a randomized, blinded study. All patients had been stabilized and had showed moderate improvement in symptoms with open lamotrigine treatment by the time of randomization. The advantage of lamotrigine over placebo was more marked in patients with bipolar II than in patients with bipolar I disorder. A principal outcome difference was that relapse rates of patients taking placebo were lower for patients with bipolar I than in patients with bipolar II disorder. Because bipolar I disorder is defined by a full manic episode, whereas bipolar II disorder is defined by a full depressive episode plus hypomania, the results suggest that the benefits of the therapeutic relationship in the placebo-assigned patients were largely evident in the bipolar I patients, who were more at risk for manic relapse, rather than in the bipolar II patients, who were more at risk for depressive relapse.

Neither the Bowden et al. nor the Calabrese et al. study was designed to test the point, but each serves to frame questions whose answers should clarify the benefits that may accrue from psychosocial interventions in bipolar disorder and what the practicing clinician can expect from supportive or more specific psychotherapies.

Support groups, particularly those organized through local chapters of the National Depressive and Manic-Depressive Association, offer substantial benefits to patients with bipolar disorder. These groups can also help patients deal with demoralization from the social consequences of their illness, because patients who have coped successfully with their own illnesses can provide practical suggestions and serve as positive role models.

Pharmacotherapy

General Considerations

Firm evidence-based guidelines for maintenance treatment of bipolar disorder are inherently difficult to establish. The best data come from placebo-controlled studies. However, it is impractical and ethically questionable to enroll patients with more severe illness histories into long-term studies in which placebo monotherapy is one of the treatments. Thus, although placebo-controlled data provide conclusive evidence of efficacy, they have limitations in generalizability to the full spectrum of bipolar disorder (Baldessarini et al. 2000; Bowden et al. 2000). Therefore, active comparative trials and open trials must be turned to as the basis for treatment recommendations.

Studies indicate that the largest differences among mood stabilizer treatments for bipolar disorder generally occur in the first 6 months of treatment (Bowden et al. 2000; Coryell et al. 1997). Beyond that point, the rates of new episodes or marked changes in symptoms change little across treatments. This can be expected because to stay in a treatment for a prolonged period, a patient must at least be tolerant of the treatment and avoid major symptoms.

Medications with excellent tolerability are crucial. Otherwise, unpleasant side effects contribute to poor adherence to the treatment regimen. Adherence is often facilitated by cautious dosage reduction. Any medication shown to have a destabilizing effect on the patient should be tapered and discontinued as soon as its short-term use is concluded. This applies categorically to currently approved antidepressant medications. There is some evidence that such destabilizing risk is greater with tricyclic antidepressants than with serotonin reuptake inhibitors or bupropion.

A high percentage of patients with bipolar disorder have psychotic symptoms when experiencing mania. In addition, there is evidence that a psychotic dimension, composed of delusional thought and impaired insight, is one of a small number of primary behavioral dimensions of bipolar disorder (Swann et al. 1999). There is inferential evidence that a minority of patients with bipolar disorder may need to take an antipsychotic medication indefinitely to control behavioral symptoms that otherwise contribute to full manic episodes (Sachs 1996). There is strong evidence from well-designed studies of acute mania that treatments with atypical antipsychotics, specifically olanzapine and risperidone, combined with lithium or valproate, may provide greater improvement in mania than occurs with lithium or valproate alone (Sachs and Ghaemi 2000; Tohen et al. 2000b). Open studies and case series suggest that other combination treatments with mood stabilizers involving the use of adjunctive medications are also more efficacious than monotherapy regimens.

Valproate

Two randomized studies provide evidence for the efficacy of valproate in maintenance treatment of bipolar disorder. Lambert and Venaud (1992) compared valpromide, an amide form of valproate, with lithium in 150 patients during an 18-month period. New episode rates were 20% lower among valpromide-treated than lithium-treated patients, and tolerability was somewhat better for valpromide-treated patients. The study is limited by an open design and inclusion of recurrent unipolar depressed patients as well as bipolar patients.

In the other randomized study, Bowden et al. (2000) indicated that the time it took for half the patients to experience a recurrence of a manic or depressive episode was 46% greater with divalproex sodium treatment than placebo treatment, and greater with divalproex sodium than with lithium. The most beneficial effect of divalproex sodium was the longer time it took for divalproex sodium–treated patients to experience a recurrent manic episode (Table 4–2). The percentage of patients completing the year of study was 46% greater with divalproex sodium than placebo. The rates of dropout for intolerance were higher in patients treated with divalproex sodium than those treated with placebo. Thus, in all respects, divalproex sodium produced favorable results. The magnitude of advantage of divalproex sodium over placebo was greater among patients who had been treated with divalproex sodium during the acute manic episode before randomization. The study is limited by having randomized patients with a relatively less severe form of bipolar I disorder, possibly having employed higher than necessary dosages of both drugs, and failure to achieve a significant difference among the treatment groups on the planned primary variable. The study does provide strong evidence of the maintenance-phase effectiveness of divalproex sodium in patients who achieved remission of manic symptoms with divalproex sodium while experiencing acute mania.

A prospective, open-label study of valproate in patients with rapid-cycling bipolar disorder indicated moderate sustained benefit on depressive symptoms and marked benefit on manic symptoms (Calabrese and Delucchi 1990). In a prospective study of rapid-cycling patients on open treatment with the combination of divalproex sodium and lithium, Calabrese et al. (2000) found that a high percentage of patients achieved remission of manic symptomatology. However, a much lower percentage achieved remission of depressive symptomatology, despite less stringent requirements for improvement in depression than mania. This observation has potentially important implications for clinicians. The data strongly suggest that treatments other than divalproex sodium alone, lithium alone, or the two combined are needed for depressive components of the illness in rapid-cycling patients.

Table 4–2. Time to recurrence in a 1-year randomized trial of divalproex sodium, lithium, or placebo in patients with bipolar I disorder

Relapse time	Divalproex sodium (n = 187)	Lithium (n = 91)	Placebo (n = 94)
	Treatment group		
Time to 50% relapse with any mood episode, d (95% CL)	275 (167, NC)	189 (88, NC)	173 (101, NC)
Time to 25% relapse with mania, d (95% CL)	> 365 (NC)	293 (71, NC)	189 (84, NC)
Time to 25% relapse with depression, d (95% CL)	126 (100, 204)	81 (33, 234)	101 (55, 190)

Note. Values are presented as no. (%) unless otherwise indicated. CL = confidence limits; NC = not calculable.

Source. Adapted with permission from Bowden CL, Calabrese JR, McElroy SL, et al.: "A Randomized, Placebo-Controlled 12-Month Trial of Divalproex and Lithium in Treatment of Outpatients With Bipolar I Disorder." *Archives of General Psychiatry* 57:481–489, 2000. Copyright 2000, American Medical Association.

Lithium

Early studies provide strong evidence of reduced rates of relapse with lithium as monotherapy or in combination with a variety of other treatments, including electroconvulsive therapy (ECT) (Coppen et al. 1971). These early studies have been criticized as having inflated relapse rates in the placebo-assigned groups, because patients were abruptly terminated from stable doses of lithium at the point of randomization (Moncrieff 1995). Another randomized, open comparison of lithium versus carbamazepine has been completed (Greil et al. 1997). Lithium was somewhat more efficacious and better tolerated than carbamazepine. The differences were principally observable when broader criteria of treatment efficacy were employed. For example, looking at the development of a new episodes, hospitalizations, or requirements for an additional medication provided more sensitive measures and indicators of greater difference between the treatments than did assessment of time to new episodes alone.

The three randomized maintenance studies of the past decade all suggest that the time remaining in treatment, completion of a planned period of treatment, and rates of treatment dropout regardless of cause are statistically stronger measures than measures of time to full episodes. We recommend that these indices be used by investigators in future clinical research assessments. It seems likely that attention to such indices in clinical practice is also justified, regardless of the particular regimen. Strong evidence exists that treatment discontinuation is associated per se with increased likelihood of relapse and that costs of treatment increase dramatically with discontinuation. Such a focus assumes greater importance of patient welfare and the costs associated with the illness.

Open naturalistic studies in the 1990s consistently indicated relatively low rates of treatment continuation and only marginally good outcomes with lithium therapy (Coryell et al. 1997; Gitlin et al. 1995; Harrow et al. 1990; Maj et al. 1998; Vestergaard et al. 1998). However, a subset of patients clearly did well for years, and persistence with lithium treatment was associated with rates of suicide and suicidal behaviors lower than rates observed among patients with untreated bipolar disorder. The low rates of good outcome were substantially associated with the low tolerability of lithium and the resulting patient discontinuation of the drug. Certain features of bipolar disorder may be predictive of good long-term outcomes. Unfortunately, in many instances, it is unclear whether these outcomes are associated with the course of the illness per se or with lithium therapy. Table 4–3 presents bipolar disorder features predictive of poor long-term response in patients treated with lithium and lists medications shown to improve response.

Notably, in three blinded randomized studies (Bowden et al. 2000; Denicoff et al. 1997; Dunner et al. 1976), lithium was associated with improvement in manic symptomatology, but depressive symptomatology worsened. Early randomized maintenance studies and more recent open naturalistic studies of lithium did not distinguish outcomes by type of episode (i.e., depressive versus hypomanic or manic). Despite the view that lithium may have antidepressant effects, the results warrant close attention to possible development of depressive symptoms in the course of continued lithium treatment and raise the possibility that either dosage reduction or change to an alternative mood stabilizer is a reasonable option if depressive symptoms persist.

Table 4–3. Predictors of poor long-term response in patients treated with lithium and medications shown to improve response

	Medications shown to improve response	Reference(s)
Atypical mania	Carbamazepine, divalproex sodium	Greil et al. 1998; Calabrese et al. 1992
Greater severity of illness	None	
Many previous episodes, especially depression	None	
Rapid cycling	Valproate; combined lithium and carbamazepine; combined lithium, carbamazepine, and valproate	Denicoff et al. 1997
Substance abuse	Divalproex sodium	Brady and Sonne 1995

There is clear evidence that abrupt discontinuation of lithium worsens short-term illness course. Clinicians need to emphasize this risk to patients taking lithium for maintenance treatment of bipolar disorder, because treatment discontinuation is a result of a) severe adverse effects of the medication and b) patient's risk-taking behavior and their desire to consider themselves cured or able to cope with the illness without medication.

As with divalproex sodium, dosing and serum level guidelines for lithium are less well established for maintenance treatment than for treatment of mania. Gelenberg et al. (1989) reported better outcomes among patients with serum levels between 0.8 and 1.0 mEq/L than for patients with serum levels between 0.4 and 0.6. However, the higher relapse rates of patients whose levels were in the lower range were largely limited to the subset of patients whose dosages at randomization were reduced from higher levels clinically associated with favorable response. The subset of patients whose prestudy serum lithium levels were in the 0.4 to 0.6 mEq/L range had equally good outcomes, whether randomized to the high or the low serum range. Maj et al. (1998)

reported that patients with levels consistently above 0.5 mEq/L had lower rates of rehospitalization than prior to treatment. Acknowledging the inadequacy of the evidence, we continue patients at serum lithium levels less than 0.8 mEq/L or valproate serum levels less than 45 µg/mL if they have benefited from either medication but have experienced adverse effects that interfere with their function and general medical health or appear unwilling to take the medication faithfully.

Lamotrigine

Lamotrigine is a new component in our growing armamentarium. Lamotrigine has been reported to be effective for up to 48 weeks both as a monotherapy and add-on therapy in patients with bipolar I or bipolar II disorder (Calabrese et al. 1999). A subsequent 26-week randomized, double-blind, placebo-controlled study of lamotrigine in patients with rapid-cycling bipolar disorder indicated significantly greater efficacy than placebo on most outcome measures (Calabrese et al. 2000). In particular, lamotrigine was associated with greater likelihood that the patient would complete the study without additional medication. The study suggests greater advantage of lamotripine use in the subset of patients with bipolar II than bipolar I disorder. This is of interest because bipolar II disorder is characterized by full depressive episodes and hypomania, rather than mania as in bipolar I disorder, therefore suggesting that the benefit may have principally been on or linked to the depressive psychopathology. These data, along with evidence that lamotrigine is effective in treating acute bipolar depression but not mania, provide strong evidence that lamotrigine has mood-stabilizing properties principally or solely effective on the depressive component of bipolar disorder. Unlike standard antidepressant medications, lamotrigine has not been associated with increased rates of cycling or manic symptoms in patients studied in placebo-controlled trials. Lamotrigine does not cause weight gain and has a benign adverse effect profile, with headache as the only side effect, which occurs more commonly in drug-treated than placebo-treated patients. The medication can cause severe rash of the erythema multiformae, Stevens Johnson vasculitis type. Higher incidences occurred in early epilepsy trials, in which lamotrigine was started at doses of 100 mg/day or higher. Risk of serious rash is lower when clinicians prescribe a gradually increasing dosage. The most recent data indicate a rate of less than 1 patient per 1,000. Lamotrigine is metabolized by glucuronidation, which is how valproate is principally metabolized. Concurrent use of the two drugs requires slower initial dosage escalation of lamotrigine and, sometimes, lower steady state dosage than would be used in monotherapy.

Carbamazepine

The effectiveness of carbamazepine in prophylactic treatment of bipolar disorder remains unclear (Post et al. 1997). In a randomized, open 2½-year study, Greil et al. (1997) found lithium to be superior to carbamazepine on most outcome measures. Carbamazepine was somewhat more effective than lithium in patients with atypical forms of manic episodes (Greil et al. 1998). Two crossover studies of treatment with lithium, carbamazepine, or both reported that combined therapy with the two medications yielded a higher proportion of sustained functional improvement than either treatment alone (Denicoff et al. 1997; Stromgren 1990). The dermatologic, neuromuscular, and cognitive side effects of carbamazepine are largely associated with dosage escalation. Therefore, patients who become stabilized on carbamazepine often have fewer side effects than acutely treated patients.

Antipsychotic Medications

A substantial percentage of patients with bipolar disorder are treated adjunctively with antipsychotic medications. The results of one placebo-controlled study of prophylactic treatment with an antipsychotic, flupenthixol, were negative (Esparon et al. 1986). The well-known adverse side-effect profile of traditional antipsychotics has limited studies of their use in maintenance treatment of bipolar disorder. Several open case reports and one randomized open study of clozapine in combination with usual care versus usual care alone indicated benefits from clozapine during maintenance treatment (Suppes et al. 1999). Atypical antipsychotic drugs have fewer or no extrapyramidal side effects, do not appear to worsen depressive symptoms, and have lower anticholinergic properties than traditional antipsychotics. These agents must also be considered part of the new armamentarium available to clinicians.

Olanzapine has been approved for treatment of mania, and both olanzapine and risperidone combined with lithium or valproate have shown greater efficacy in treating patients with acute mania than either mood stabilizer alone (Tohen et al. 1999). Therefore, there is increased interest in these medications in the long-term treatment of bipolar disorder, but no randomized controlled studies have been published. When psychotic symptoms or hostility and irritability are prominent long-term symptoms of bipolar disorder, atypical antipsychotic medications are reasonable considerations for adjunctive therapy. The mean dosage of olanzapine used in studies of mania has been approximately 12 mg/day, and for risperidone approximately 6 mg/day.

Other Treatments

The current interest in a variety of other treatments for bipolar disorder, including topiramate, gabapentin, omega-3 fatty acids, and inositol, has been largely generated by case studies in mania. There are insufficient data to recommend use of any of these drugs. An open trial of topiramate added to current therapy in 54 bipolar patients for 10 weeks reported evidence of improvement among patients entering with manic, mixed, or cycling presentations, but little improvement for patients entering with depressed or euthymic presentations (McElroy et al. 2000). Results of placebo-controlled studies of topiramate and gabapentin in acutely manic patients have been negative. Topiramate is also of interest because of its contributions toward reduced appetite and weight loss, a potentially useful attribute given the tendency of several treatments for bipolar disorder to increase appetite and weight.

Combination Treatment

Bipolar disorder is inherently a multifactorial condition. In addition to manic and depressive symptoms, patients may have anxiety states, irritability, psychotic symptoms, comorbid attention-deficit symptoms, and clinically significant sleep disturbances. There is increasing evidence, largely from naturalistic studies, that a majority of bipolar patients will achieve better symptomatic and functional outcomes with some form of combined treatment (Denicoff et al. 1997; Solomon et al. 1997). It is advisable to commence maintenance treatment with as few medications as possible. However, dimensions of the illness that remain inadequately managed with simpler regimens warrant additional medications and a sufficient trial duration to assess whether benefits are maintained. Furthermore, it may be possible to reduce the dosage of a medication to a better-tolerated level when drugs are combined, in contrast to the dosage employed in a monotherapy regimen.

Summary

Bipolar disorder is the prototype of an episodic, recurrent psychiatric disorder, creating havoc among its patients when untreated. During the latter half of the 20th century, we made terrific progress in learning how to reduce and modulate recurrences and their destructive consequences. Limitations in available treatments created ongoing problems for patients, families, and clinicians, however. During the past decade, our treatment portfolio has expanded considerably, and rapidly growing data reveal that we can do much more for those with bipolar disorder. Treatment success depends on a multifactorial approach and frequently requires combination pharmacotherapy, sometimes combining the "old" with the "new." As the "new" continues to expand, there is reason for optimism.

References

American Psychiatric Association: Diagnostic and Statistical Manual of Mental Disorders, 4th Edition, Text Revision. Washington, DC, American Psychiatric Association, 2000

Baldessarini RJ, Tohen M, Tondo L: Maintenance treatment in bipolar disorder (comment). Arch Gen Psychiatry 57:490–492, 2000

Bowden CL, Calabrese JR, McElroy SL, et al: A randomized, placebo-controlled 12-month trial of divalproex and lithium in treatment of outpatients with bipolar I disorder. Arch Gen Psychiatry 57:481–489, 2000

Brady KT, Sonne SC: The relationship between substance abuse and bipolar disorder. J Clin Psychiatry 56 (3, suppl):19–24, 1995

Calabrese JR, Delucchi GA: Spectrum of efficacy of valproate in 55 patients with rapid-cycling bipolar disorder. Am J Psychiatry 147:431–434, 1990

Calabrese JR, Markovitz PJ, Kimmel SE, et al: Spectrum of efficacy of valproate in 78 rapid-cycling bipolar patients. J Clin Psychopharmacol 12:535–565, 1992

Calabrese JR, Bowden CL, Sachs GS, et al: A double-blind placebo-controlled study of lamotrigine monotherapy in outpatients with bipolar I depression. J Clin Psychiatry 60:79–88, 1999

Calabrese JR, Suppes T, Bowden CL, et al: A double-blind, placebo-controlled, prophylaxis study of lamotrigine in rapid-cycling bipolar disorder. J Clin Psychiatry 61:841–850, 2000

Coppen A, Noguera R, Bailey J, et al: Prophylactic lithium in affective disorders. Lancet 2:275–279, 1971

Coryell W, Winokur G, Solomon D, et al: Lithium and recurrence in a long-term follow-up of bipolar affective disorder. Psychol Med 27:281–289, 1997

Denicoff KD, Smith-Jackson EE, Disney ER, et al: Comparative prophylactic efficacy of lithium, carbamazepine, and the combination in bipolar disorder. J Clin Psychiatry 58:470–478, 1997

Dunner DL, Stallone F, Fieve RR: Lithium carbonate and affective disorders, V: a double-blind study of prophylaxis of depression in bipolar illness. Arch Gen Psychiatry 33:117–120, 1976

Esparon J, Kolloori J, Naylor GJ, et al: Comparison of the prophylactic action of flupenthixol with placebo in lithium treated manic-depressive patients. Br J Psychiatry 148:723–725, 1986

Evans DA, Nemeroff CB: The dexamethasone suppression test in mixed bipolar disorder. Am J Psychiatry 140:615–617, 1983

Frank E, Kupfer DJ, Ehlers CJ, et al: Interpersonal and social rhythm therapy for bipolar disorder: integrating interpersonal and behavioral approaches. Behavioral Therapist 17:143–149, 1994

Garvey MJ, Hwang S, Teubner-Rhodes D, et al: Dextroamphetamine treatment of mania. J Clin Psychiatry 48:412–413, 1987

Gelenberg AJ, Kane JM, Keller MB, et al: Comparison of standard and low serum levels of lithium for maintenance treatment of bipolar disorder. N Engl J Med 321:1489–1493, 1989

Gitlin MJ, Swendsen J, Heller TL, et al: Relapse and impairment in bipolar disorder. Am J Psychiatry 152:1635–1640, 1995

Goodwin FK, Jamison KR: Manic-Depressive Illness. New York, Oxford University Press, 1990

Greil W, Ludwig-Mayerhofer W, Erazo N, et al: Lithium versus carbamazepine in the maintenance treatment of bipolar disorders—a randomized study. J Affect Disord 43:151–161, 1997

Greil W, Kleindienst N, Erazo N, et al: Differential response to lithium and carbamazepine in the prophylaxis of bipolar disorder. J Clin Psychopharmacol 18:455–460, 1998

Harrow M, Goldberg JF, Grossman LS, et al: Outcome in manic disorders: a naturalistic follow-up study. Arch Gen Psychiatry 47:665–671, 1990

Hirschfeld R, Weisler R, Keck P Jr, et al: Cost-effectiveness evaluation of divalproex sodium vs. lithium in the treatment of bipolar disorder, in 1999 New Research Program and Abstracts, American Psychiatric Association 152nd Annual Meeting, Washington, DC, May 15–20, 1999. Washington, DC, American Psychiatric Association, 1999, p 262

Horgan D: Change of diagnosis to manic depressive illness. Psychol Med 11:517–523, 1981

Jamison KR: An Unquiet Mind. New York, Alfred Knopf, 1995

Johnson RE, McFarland BH: Lithium use and discontinuation in a health maintenance organization. Am J Psychiatry 153:993–1000, 1996

Krishnan RR, Maltbie AA, Davidson JR: Abnormal cortisol suppression in bipolar patients with simultaneous manic and depressive symptoms. Am J Psychiatry 140:203–205, 1983

Lambert PA, Venaud G: Comparative study of valpromide versus lithium as prophylactic treatment in affective disorders. Nervure 5:57–65, 1992

Maj M, Pirozzi R, Magliano L, et al: Long-term outcome of lithium prophylaxis in bipolar disorder: A 5-year prospective study of 402 patients at a lithium clinic. Am J Psychiatry 155:30–35, 1998

McElroy SL, Suppes T, Keck PE Jr, et al: Open-label adjunctive topiramate in the treatment of bipolar disorders. Biol Psychiatry 47:1025–1033, 2000

Miklowitz DJ, Goldstein MJ: Behavioral family treatment for patients with bipolar affective disorder. Behav Modif 14:457–489, 1990

Moncrieff J: Lithium revisited. A re-examination of the placebo-controlled trials of lithium prophylaxis in manic-depressive disorder (editorial). Br J Psychiatry 167:569–573, 1995

Nemeroff CB: The neurobiology of depression. Sci Am 278:42–49, 1998

Post RM, Denicoff KD, Frye MA, et al: Re-evaluating carbamazepine prophylaxis in bipolar disorder. Br J Psychiatry 170:202–204, 1997

Sachs GS: Bipolar mood disorder: practical strategies for acute and maintenance phase treatment. J Clin Psychopharmacol 16 (2 suppl 1): 32S-47S, 1996

Sachs G, Ghaemi SN: Efficacy and tolerability of risperidone versus placebo in combination with lithium or valproate in acute mania (abstract). Eur Neuropsychopharmacol 10 (suppl 3): S240, 2000

Silverstone T, Romans S, Hunt N, et al: Is there a seasonal pattern of relapse in bipolar affective disorders? A dual northern and southern hemisphere cohort study. Br J Psychiatry 167:58–60, 1995

Solomon DA, Ryan CE, Keitner GI, et al: A pilot study of lithium carbonate plus divalproex sodium for the continuation and maintenance treatment of patients with bipolar I disorder. J Clin Psychiatry 58:95–99, 1997

Stromgren LS: The combination of lithium and carbamazepine in treatment and prevention of manic-depressive disorder: A review and a case report. Compr Psychiatry 31:261–265, 1990

Suppes T, Webb A, Paul B, et al: Clinical outcome in a randomized 1-year trial of clozapine versus treatment as usual for patients with treatment-resistant illness and a history of mania. Am J Psychiatry 156: 1164–1169, 1999

Swann AC, Secunda SK, Stokes PE, et al: Stress, depression, and mania: relationship between perceived role of stressful events and clinical and biochemical characteristics. Acta Psychiatr Scand 81:389–397, 1990

Swann AC, Bowden CL, Calabrese JR, et al: Differential effect of number of previous episodes of affective disorder on response to lithium or divalproex in acute mania. Am J Psychiatry 156:1264–1266, 1999

Tohen M, Sanger TM, McElroy SL, et al: Olanzapine versus placebo in the treatment of acute mania. Am J Psychiatry 156:702–709, 1999

Tohen M, Hennen J, Zarate CM Jr, et al: Two-year syndromal and functional recovery in 219 cases of first-episode major affective disorder with psychotic features. Am J Psychiatry 157:220–228, 2000a

Tohen M, Jacobs TG, Grundy SL, et al: Efficacy of olanzapine in acute bipolar mania: a double-blind, placebo-controlled study. Arch Gen Psychiatry 57:841-849, 2000b

Vestergaard P, Licht RW, Brodersen A, et al: Outcome of lithium prophylaxis: a prospective follow-up of affective disorder patients assigned to high and low serum lithium levels. Acta Psychiatr Scand 98:310–315, 1998

Chapter 5

New Depression Treatment Strategies

What Does the Future Hold for Therapeutic Uses of Minimally Invasive Brain Stimulation?

Mark S. George, M.D.
Ziad Nahas, M.D.
Xing-Bao Li, M.D.
Jeong-Ho Chae, M.D.
Nicholas Oliver, B.S.
Arif Najib, B.S.
Berry Anderson, R.N.

In the 1980s, a new era dawned as psychiatrists and neurologists discovered new tools for functional brain imaging, including positron emission tomography (PET). For the first time, one could look, noninvasively, and observe the brain at work and rest, in health and disease. Many predicted that these tools would transform the clinical neurosciences, particularly psychiatry, even perhaps eliminating the need for clinical diagnostic interviews. Now, 20 years later, functional brain imaging tools have greatly informed our understanding of the brain. They have helped destigmatize

Some of the studies discussed in this review were funded in part by grants from or research collaborations with Dupont Pharma, Cyberonics, Medtronic, the National Alliance for Research on Schizophrenia and Depression (NARSAD), the Stanley Foundation, and National Institute of Neurological Disorders and Stroke (NINDS) RO1 NS40956–01.

neuropsychiatric illnesses. However, with only a few notable examples (e.g., multiple sclerosis and acute stroke management), the diagnosis and management of most neuropsychiatric disorders have not been greatly affected by advances in brain imaging techniques.

Psychiatrists still do not order brain imaging tests for diagnosis of depression, except for the occasional scan to exclude a brain tumor or stroke as the causative disease. Why? To date, there has not been a consensus on which brain regions change during an episode of depression. Many studies have found decreased resting activity in the prefrontal cortex with associated limbic hypoactivity. However, these findings are neither specific to depression (Dolan et al. 1993) nor present in all cases (Drevets et al. 1992) in a magnitude that allows one to use imaging as a clinical tool for depression diagnosis or management (Nahas et al. 1998). Further, the diagnosis of depression as currently classified is straightforward with a competent clinical examination and history. In addition, most pharmacological and behavioral treatments for depression work regardless of whether the depression is primary or secondary to another illness such as a brain tumor or stroke. Thus, in the absence of the need to refine diagnoses to maximize treatment, there has not been a push to develop imaging paradigms for better understanding of different disease pathogeneses that may underlie depressive symptoms. Nevertheless, some provocative imaging studies have shown clear differences in regional brain activity in different subsets of depression. For example, late-onset depression is associated with more white matter disease than depression that occurs early in life (Coffey et al. 1988, 1989). Resting brain scans have distinguished patients with bipolar depression from patients with unipolar depression (Breitner et al. 1990) and have indicated which depressed patients will respond to sleep deprivation (Ebert et al. 1991, 1994; Wu et al. 1992), fluoxetine (Mayberg et al. 1997), electroconvulsive therapy (ECT) (Nobler et al. 1994), or transcranial magnetic stimulation (TMS) (Teneback et al. 1999). Moreover, imaging studies in patients with long-remitted depression can even discern those who will experience a temporary relapse with a pharmacological depletion paradigm (Bremner et al. 1997).

With this ever-expanding body of studies, one might wonder why functional neuroimaging has not had more of an impact in clinical settings of depression diagnosis and management. One reason might be that the debut of many of these new imaging tools coincided with the emergence of stringent cost-containment measures in all areas of medicine, particularly in mental health. Thus, these tools were never placed in large clinical settings where their clinical use could slowly emerge. Further, the revolution in pharmacology has proceeded at a breathtaking pace, and these developments have been independent of a need for more detailed regional neurobiology. Thus, if most people with depression respond to medications with few side effects, the momentum is not generated for more detailed understanding of disease pathogenesis and regional neurobiology. Thus, there has not been a real clinical demand pushing research in this area. The new brain stimulation technologies discussed in this chapter may drastically change this.

An important factor behind the development of brain stimulation techniques that build on neuroimaging involves the notion of efficient delivery of therapeutics. Theoretically, giving an oral medication is one of the least efficient ways to change activity in specific brain regions. The pill must be absorbed by the gut and travel throughout the body, where a small portion of it is transported across the blood-brain barrier. There, the medication travels throughout the entire brain, with only some of it reaching its intended target circuit or region. Thus, there is potential for side effects in the periphery and in the brain through unintended exposure. The more discrete the placement of a drug or intervention, the more effective it will be and the fewer side effects will occur. For example, some effective antidepressants, such as thyrotropin releasing hormone (TRH), are marginally effective when given peripherally (by mouth or intravenously). However they have potent, but transient, antidepressant effects when injected intrathecally directly into the central nervous system (Marangell et al. 1997). The minimally invasive brain stimulation (MIBS) strategies discussed in this chapter have the potential to change local pharmacology without unintended bodily side effects in ways that oral medications cannot.

In addition to the advancing knowledge of neuropsychiatric circuits, another factor driving the development of MIBS techniques is the fact that available medications do not work for all patients with depression. Thus, in patients with treatment-resistant depression, there has been a push for more aggressive somatic interventions. In the last century, these interventions consisted of brain surgery and ECT. We are now at the threshold of launching a new group of therapeutic tools (designated MIBS in this chapter) that build on the knowledge of functional circuits that has accumulated over the past 20 years (Table 5–1). Knowledge of the pathological circuits involved in some neuropsychiatric disorders, such as Parkinson's disease and obsessive-compulsive disorder, is expanding. These disorders will likely be at the forefront of the revolution in the use of MIBS techniques to treat neuropsychiatric illnesses. In this chapter, we focus on how knowledge about the specific brain regions involved in depression and mood regulation is rapidly expanding and setting the stage for use of these new brain stimulation techniques. These new techniques offer the promise of revolutionizing the understanding and treatment of depression. Each technique will need to be evaluated to determine if it is effective in preventing recurrences of depression, singly or in combination with other treatments. However, it must be remembered that this new field is in its infancy and that all of the techniques that follow, except ECT, are considered experimental and are not available in the United States for clinical work.

Electroconvulsive Therapy

Early in the 20th century, Von Meduna in Italy was the first to consider ECT—the oldest and best-proven brain stimulation technique—as a potential therapeutic treatment. His interest was based on faulty clinical observations that patients with schizophrenia had no seizures and that patients with epilepsy were not psychotic. (Subsequent studies have shown that both these observations are likely to be false.) Meduna, and then researchers in the United States, produced generalized seizures in patients with psychosis, some of whom improved (probably those with psychotic depression). Initial studies were done using chemical injections to

Table 5–1. Current and potential somatic interventions for the treatment of severe depression

Somatic intervention	Regional specificity	Clinical applicability	Invasiveness
Electroconvulsive therapy (ECT)	+	++++	+++ Requires anesthesia, causes generalized seizure
Magnetic seizure therapy (MST)	++	+ Initial trial under way	+++ Requires anesthesia, causes generalized seizure
Transcranial electrical stimulation (TES)	+	++	++ May cause scalp irritation
Transcranial magnetic stimulation (TMS)	++++	+++ Clinical trials under way	+ May be painful at high intensities
Vagus nerve stimulation (VNS)	++	+++ Used for treatment of epilepsy, clinical trials for depression under way	+++ Requires surgery for pulse-generator implant
Deep brain stimulation (DBS)	+++	+++ Approved in U.S. for treatment of movement disorders and pain syndromes, no work in depression yet	++++ Requires brain surgery

Note. Plus signs represent a scale from + = minimal to ++++ = marked.

induce seizures. Studies of chemically induced convulsions and, later, ECT convulsions catalyzed the clinical winnowing of applications to the current use profile of ECT for mood disorders and occasionally for catatonia and Parkinson's disease. For reviews of the history of ECT, see Impastato (1960) and Lisanby and Sackeim (2000).

The history of ECT demonstrates its overapplication to many conditions, with clinical use delineating both the clinical applications in which it is effective and the modes of application that improve its efficacy (e.g., dose titration). For example, ECT was used for 30 years before it was determined that prefrontal, not parietal, application of the electrodes was necessary for a therapeutic antidepressant effect, regardless of whether a generalized seizure occurred (Sackeim et al. 1993). Only in the 1990s did we learn that although a generalized convulsion is necessary to treat depression, it is not sufficient and must be induced with electrodes over the prefrontal cortex. Similarly, we have learned that dose titration drastically improves antidepressant efficacy and that the width of the commonly used ECT current pulse is extremely inefficient (and toxic) from a neurobiologic standpoint of what is needed to depolarize neurons. High-intensity, ultra-brief–pulse, right-unilateral prefrontal ECT has similar efficacy to bilateral ECT (Sackeim et al. 2000).

Using single photon emission computed tomography (SPECT) and more recently PET scans, Nobler et al. (1994, 2000) found that patients who responded to ECT had a greater reduction in prefrontal blood flow immediately following ECT. Thus, there appears to be anatomic specificity for where the ECT stimulus is most needed and most effective. Unfortunately, the skull acts as a large resistor when electrical current is applied to the scalp; therefore, the bulk of the energy of an ECT pulse does not go directly into brain and the electrical energy of ECT cannot be focused.

These findings help convey the excitement and revival of interest in ECT theory and practice. In another important development, Lisanby and Sackeim succeeded in using powerful alternating *magnetic* (not electrical) fields to cause seizures in primates (Lisanby et al. 1998a, 1998b, in press). This technique is called magnetic seizure therapy (MST). Unlike electricity, magnetic fields pass unimpeded through the skull and soft tissue and thus can be applied in a more focused manner. This development opens up the possibility of inducing ECT-like seizures in humans with a magnetic field, likely reducing greatly the cognitive side effects that probably result from unnecessary passage of electrical current in ancillary brain regions during standard ECT.

Lisanby, Schlaepfer, and Sackeim (2000) reported that MST is feasible in humans. The authors produced magnetic-induced seizures on three different mornings in a woman undergoing a course of conventional ECT for the treatment of depression. Although these developments are exciting and offer the potential for a new form of therapy, they should be viewed with some caution. In this woman, the seizures were induced over the motor cortex, which is the easiest brain region in which to generate a seizure. Current theories of ECT mechanisms of action would predict that the seizure needs to start in the prefrontal cortex, and this will likely require newer, more powerful machines than the one used for the proof-of-concept demonstration. Most important, efficacy and side effects of MST are not known. Thus, ECT may be further refined to better direct the origin of the seizure and spare other brain regions. However, recent developments with all other MIBS techniques—nonconvulsive transcranial magnetic stimulation (TMS), vagus nerve stimulation (VNS), and deep brain stimulation (DBS)—challenge the doctrine that a generalized convulsion is necessary to produce an antidepressant effect (George and Wassermann 1994; George et al. 1999b).

Transcranial Magnetic Stimulation

TMS, a noninvasive method for modifying regional brain activity, uses a powerful hand-held magnet to create a time-varying magnetic field. When placed on the scalp, this powerful magnetic field creates electrical currents in the superficial cortex—a form of electrodeless electrical stimulation (Figure 5–1). Thus, TMS can depolarize cortical neurons and cause downstream changes in connected brain regions. For reviews of TMS, see George and Belmaker (2000) and George et al. (1999a).

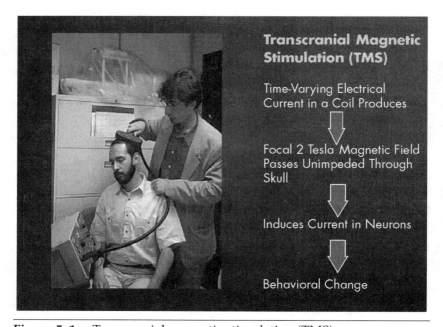

Figure 5–1. Transcranial magnetic stimulation (TMS).
Ziad Nahas, M.D., demonstrates the TMS technique on Ananda Shastri, Ph.D.
Note the capacitor (lower left), which sends electrical energy through a coil of
wire that rests on the scalp (with electrical insulation). The powerful but brief
electrical current creates a transient magnetic field that passes unencumbered
through the skull and creates electrical currents within the brain.

The magnetic field produced by modern TMS devices has a
transient (microseconds) strength of about 1.0 to 1.5 tesla and can
activate neurons 1.5–2.0 cm from the surface of the coil (Bohning
2000). If TMS pulses are delivered repetitively and rhythmically,
the procedure is called repetitive TMS (rTMS). Modern machines
allow transcranial magnetic stimuli to be delivered extremely
fast, faster than once per second (1 Hz). This is called high-frequency
or fast rTMS (>1 Hz). Currently, there are four commercial manufac-
turers of TMS machines: Cadwell, Dantec-Medtronic, Magstim, and
Neotonus.

One of the popular initial uses of TMS was to map the motor
cortex, because the effects of stimulation could easily be measured by electromyography of the motor evoked potential (MEP)
(Pascual-Leone et al. 1994d) in peripheral muscles. TMS over the

motor cortex has become a valuable tool for investigating the basic physiology of the motor cortex in health and disease (Pascual-Leone et al. 1994a; Wassermann et al. 1992). For example, TMS has been used to measure central motor conduction time in various neurological diseases, such as Parkinson's disease and multiple sclerosis, as well as to study the somatotropic organization of the motor cortex (Homberg et al. 1991; Pascual-Leone et al. 1994b, 1994c). TMS has also been widely used to measure connectivity and excitability of the cerebral cortex with various measures, such as the motor threshold, MEP input-output curve, MEP map, silent period, and paired-pulse facilitation (Reutens et al. 1993a, 1993b; Ziemann and Hallett 2000). These measurements have shown increasing relevance in clinical psychiatry research. For example, there is evidence of altered motor cortex excitability in several psychiatric disorders, which changes with certain medications, particularly anticonvulsants (Greenberg et al. 1998; Ziemann and Hallett 2000; Wassermann et al. 1998). Thus, TMS may prove to be valuable as a noninvasive diagnostic or therapeutic monitoring tool.

TMS at different frequencies and locations can cause suppression of visual perception, speech arrest, and paresthesias (Belmaker and Fleischmann 1995; Epstein et al. 1990, 1996). TMS can thus be used as a tool to map specific brain functions. Several groups have applied TMS to the study of visual information processing, language production, memory, attention, reaction time, and even more subtle brain functions, such as mood and emotion (for review, see George et al. 1999a). In sum, the ability to stimulate noninvasively and safely the brain of an awake and alert human is an important new advance in neuroscience.

For Treatment of Depression

The notion of using powerful magnetic fields to treat depression was present at the beginning of the 20th century (Beer 1902). However, it was not until 1985 that battery technology and circuits developed to the point at which TMS devices could create a magnetic field powerful enough to move the thumb when applied to the motor cortex (Barker et al. 1985). Psychiatrists initially followed the experience gained by neurologists and began by applying small doses of TMS over the vertex and motor cortex (Grisaru et al. 1994; Hoflich et al. 1993; Kolbinger et al. 1995). George and Wasserman (1994) hypothesized, from the functional imaging and ECT response data discussed previously, that large doses of subconvulsive higher frequency rTMS over the prefrontal cortex might have antidepressant effects.

As of this writing, the combined results of 16 published studies of TMS for the treatment of depression suggest that left prefrontal rTMS has acute antidepressant effects. The three initial uncontrolled clinical studies from Europe suggested, but did not prove, that single-pulse TMS applied over the vertex has antidepressant effects (Grisaru et al. 1994; Hoflich et al. 1993; Kolbinger et al. 1995). More recently, double-blind controlled studies support the efficacy of TMS in the treatment of depression. During the early 1990s, George and colleagues at the National Institute of Mental Health were the first to report that left prefrontal rTMS might be effective in the treatment of depression, first in an open study (George et al. 1995), then in a double-blind, randomized crossover study (George et al. 1997b). In the latter placebo-controlled study, 2 weeks of left prefrontal rTMS (20 Hz) had an antidepressant effect that was statistically superior to sham (placebo) stimulation, but the size of the effect was small and consisted of only a few points' reduction in the Hamilton Rating Scale for Depression (HRSD). Pascual-Leone et al. (1996b) in Spain performed a multiple placebo-controlled crossover study in 17 patients with medication-resistant psychotic depression. In a widely quoted study published in *Lancet*, Pascual-Leone et al. (1996b) reported that rTMS (10 Hz) for only 1 week on the left lateral dorsolateral prefrontal cortex resulted in a significant decrease in depressive symptoms in these patients. This study was unusual in its design of treating patients for 1 week per month at different brain regions and following them up for 6 months. Patients were on multiple medications. Although it drew much interest to the field, this clinical trial has not been replicated despite several attempts. It now appears that TMS applied in this manner takes at least several weeks to work, has more modest clinical antidepressant effects, does not work in alleviating psychotic depression, and works on the right side as well as the left. Unfortunately, the design of many early TMS depression clinical trials was based on the results of this trial. Those studies now appear to be under-powered with respect to dose and sample size.

Other open (Avery et al. 1999; Figiel et al. 1998; Triggs et al. 1999) and double-blind (Berman et al. 2000; George et al. 2000a) studies have confirmed the antidepressant effects of left prefrontal TMS, using parameters much like those used in the initial George et al. (1997b) study. However, it is highly unlikely that the parameters used in the initial George et al. (1995, 1997b) studies (e.g., frequency, intensity, pulse duration, and stimulation site of TMS) were optimal. For example, in the largest TMS study as of this writing in terms of numbers of subjects and therapeutic effect, Klein et al. (1999) found clinically significant antidepressant efficacy of slow (1 Hz) rTMS on the *right* prefrontal cortex when using a round coil.

In a more recent study, we confirmed and extended the results of these initial studies (George et al. 2000a). We studied 30 adult patients with major depression who were not taking antidepressants. Most of these patients had treatment-resistant depression. Patients were randomly assigned to a group that would receive sham (placebo) stimulation or to one of two groups that would receive active treatment (5 Hz or 20 Hz). After 2 weeks of treatment, none of the 10 patients who received placebo were classified as responders, whereas 9 of 20 patients who received active TMS had a greater than 50% drop in HRSD scores and were classified as responders. There was no significant difference in response rates between the two groups that received active treatment. Imaging studies performed on the basis of this trial showed no change in structural magnetic resonance imaging (MRI) scans before and after the 2 weeks of treatment (i.e., TMS did not cause the brain to grow or shrink or cause visible MRI changes) (Nahas et al. 2000). Further, SPECT scans showed that patients who responded to TMS had increased orbitofrontal cortex activity at baseline compared with patients who did not respond (Teneback et al. 1999) and an increase in cingulate activity after treatment compared with baseline. Following treatment, there was an even greater difference in inferior frontal blood flow in responders versus nonresponders.

Finally, MRI scans have suggested that depressed patients with a large distance from the skull to the prefrontal cortex are less likely to respond (Kozel et al. 2000) and show the least brain activation underneath the coil. This finding has led our group to question whether increased distance into the brain in older patients with depression might be the cause of the relatively weak antidepressant effects seen in these patients. We are performing MRI scans in depressed geriatric patients (see Nahas et al. 2001), measuring the distance from the skull to prefrontal cortex, and then modifying the dose of TMS to overcome this distance. An interim analysis of our open study showed that 3 out of 6 elderly depressed patients responded after 2 weeks—better than the published literature (Figiel et al. 1998). Most important, unlike the Kozel et al. (2000) study, in which age and distance were negative predictors of response using a common intensity, there was no relationship between distance into brain and response in the patients studied by Figiel and colleagues, suggesting that we are overcoming this variable with the entry scan and measurement.

Similarities between the effect and mechanism of ECT and TMS have provoked studies directly comparing the antidepressant effects of these two treatment modalities. Grunhaus et al. (1998, 2000) showed that although ECT was a more potent treatment in patients with psychotic depression, the effects of rTMS were similar to those of ECT in patients with nonpsychotic depression.

In summary, even though some negative findings for therapeutic efficacy in depressed patients have been reported (Loo et al. 1998), rTMS is a promising tool for the treatment of depression. Further studies will help determine the optimum TMS dosing strategy. It is unlikely that the initial combinations of intensity, frequency, coil shape, scalp location, number of stimuli, and dosing strategy (e.g., daily, twice daily) are optimum or even close to maximum efficacy. Improved knowledge both of the brain circuitry involved in depression and of the neurobiologic effects of TMS will help guide more effective forms of TMS. For example, it appears that more stimuli of higher intensity produce a more powerful antidepressant effect (Figure 5–2).

One of the current theories of the antidepressant effects of ECT—the anticonvulsant hypothesis of ECT—is that ECT sei-

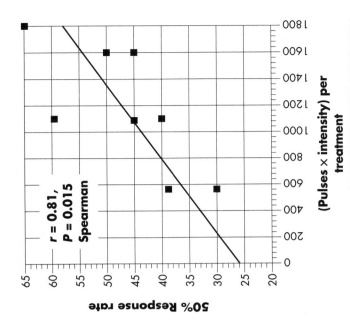

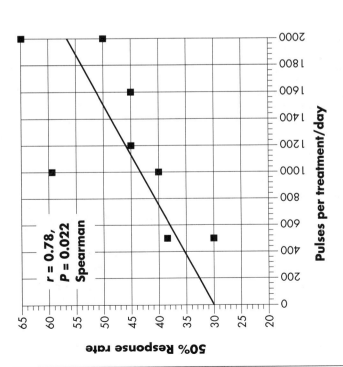

Figure 5–2. Meta-analysis of studies of transcranial magnetic stimulation (TMS) for treatment of depression.

Note. This meta-analysis suggests that current intensity parameters and doses used today may not be the most effective. HRSD = Hamilton Rating Scale for Depression; IMP = weeks after implantation; VNS = vagus nerve stimulation.

Source. Graphs compliments of Charles Epstein, M.D.

zures set into motion a cascade of events designed to stop the current seizure and prevent future seizures. Following this reasoning, ECT works by stimulating the brain's natural anticonvulsant cascade, which somehow reregulates and treats depression. If this is true, the best TMS settings for treating depression are those that also are maximally anticonvulsant. This might involve settings that take the brain to the edge of having a seizure, as George and Wassermann (1994) first proposed with fast rTMS. Alternatively, high-intensity, low-frequency TMS has shown local inhibitory effects over the motor cortex. There is a possibility that low-frequency rTMS, which seems to be safer because of its lack of proconvulsive effect, has a similar or even greater antidepressant therapeutic effect than high-frequency rTMS. This might explain the Klein et al. (1999) findings relative to the rest of the field. The magnitude of antidepressant response varies greatly across these studies. Potential reasons for this difference include stimulation at diverse intensities and frequencies, use of assorted coils, distinctive patient populations, varying concomitant medications, and degree of medication resistance. Although the literature is not entirely consistent, several trends and patterns are emerging.

In contrast to the early Pascual-Leone et al. (1996b) and Figiel et al. (1998) studies, it appears that TMS takes 2 weeks or more to achieve maximum antidepressant effect. We recommend that future TMS studies be designed for at least 3 weeks.

It appears that TMS at greater than motor threshold is more effective than TMS at less than motor threshold. Imaging studies confirm that TMS at less than motor threshold has only weak brain effects (Nahas et al. 1999b). There also appears to be a trend toward higher numbers of stimuli having greater effects. Therefore, the upper end of antidepressant effectiveness likely has not been found and is likely associated with longer (3-week) treatment with higher intensities and a greater number of stimuli.

Initial theories held that prefrontal TMS was more effective than TMS over the vertex or other sites. Although TMS functional imaging studies have clearly shown prefrontal cortex connections to important subcortical sites, only one published clinical trial has directly addressed this location issue, and it was methodologically flawed (Pascual-Leone et al. 1996b). Our recent study (George et al. 2000a) showed no striking advantage of faster stimulation (20 Hz) compared with slower (5 Hz); therefore, perhaps this was a misguided assumption that higher-frequency stimulation would have greater antidepressant efficacy. Provocative data by Kimbrell et al. (1999) suggest that the frequency of stimulation should be tailored to the baseline PET scan in terms of global hypoactivity or hyperactivity. There is also a striking lack of knowledge concerning whether a focal or more general coil should be used. Of note, the best clinical effects to date have come from a study using a round, nonfocal coil. Also unclear is whether one should use sophisticated MRI-guided devices to localize TMS focal coil placement.

Further investigations using clinical trials, brain imaging, and animal models are needed to find the best antidepressant stimulation parameters. Most important, it will be necessary to examine ways to sustain the therapeutic benefits of TMS and to identify the optimum techniques and indications for its application.

Researchers will begin to test the clinical utility of TMS as an antidepressant and the role many variables play in producing the antidepressant effect. Clinical trials will be refined and guided by findings from combining TMS with imaging and using TMS in animal models. Several groups are experimenting with methods in which TMS might be able to stimulate deeper structures, which might greatly expand its research and clinical uses.

For Treatment of Other Disorders

Several psychiatric antidepressant medications and treatments are also effective antimanic agents (e.g., anticonvulsants and ECT). In a clinical trial, Grisaru et al. (1998) found that right prefrontal TMS is antimanic compared with left prefrontal TMS. However, this result is too preliminary to draw any definite conclusions.

A pilot report that compulsive urges decreased after right lateral prefrontal rTMS (Greenberg et al. 1997) showed the potential usefulness of TMS as a probe of cortico-striato-pallido-thalamic circuits and pathophysiological processes potentially involved in the symptoms of obsessive-compulsive disorder. In addition, researchers worldwide have conducted studies on TMS in patients with schizophrenia (Hoffman et al. 1998; Nahas et al. 1999a), Parkinson's disease, Tourette's syndrome, epilepsy, and some anxiety disorders. For reviews, see George and Belmaker (2000) and George et al. (1999a).

Safety Issues and Side Effects

Although there is minimal risk of a seizure when TMS is performed within published safety guidelines, the most critical safety concern may be inadvertently causing a seizure (Lorberbaum and Wassermann 2000). In contrast to single-pulse TMS, in which seizures have not been reported in healthy persons, to date at least eight seizures have been caused by rTMS (Wassermann 1998); none have been reported in the 3 years after the published safety standards. Standard procedures for minimizing seizure risk involve excluding patients at risk for seizures, performing appropriate neurologic and laboratory examinations, properly determining the motor threshold prior to TMS, and closely monitoring patients during TMS administration for signs of potential seizure.

A muscle tension type headache and discomfort at the site of stimulation are less serious but relatively common side effects of TMS. In contrast to ECT, no deleterious cognitive effects from 2 weeks of daily slow or fast rTMS were found (Little et al. 1999). Similar to MRI, TMS can cause the movement of paramagnetic metal objects. For this reason, patients with these objects in the head or eye are generally excluded from TMS studies. TMS can cause heating of metallic implants and the inactivation of pacemakers, medication pumps, or cochlear devices. Although rTMS is an experimental procedure in the United States that requires an investigational device exemption from the U.S. Food and Drug Administration, substantial experience suggests that, at least in the short term, TMS at moderate intensity has no lasting adverse effects in adults. This is strongly supported by the Nahas et al. (2000) study, in which MRI scans were qualitatively and quantitatively assessed for structural change after TMS. This small study suggests that TMS at usual intensities and frequencies does not cause observable structural changes.

Areas of Additional Study

In addition to concerns about acute efficacy and safety, the field of TMS is beginning to address the issues of using TMS as a maintenance antidepressant treatment. Preliminary studies at our institution and at Emory University are promising in this regard. Although it is too early to tell whether TMS has long-lasting therapeutic effects, this tool has opened up possibilities for clinical exploration and treatment of psychiatric conditions. The ability to noninvasively stimulate the brain in an awake, alert human is a real advance about which neuroscientists have long dreamed. Many parameters, such as intensity, location, frequency, pulse width, intertrain interval, coil type, duration, numbers of sessions, interval between sessions, and time of day for TMS application on specific diseases, remain to be systematically explored.

It is believed that successful treatment of some psychiatric disorders is achieved by modifying neuronal activity at a systems or circuit level. TMS is able to produce immediate and longer term changes in brain circuits and thus has much potential as a therapeutic tool. As functional imaging tools continue to reveal the relevant circuitry involved in several psychiatric diseases, TMS offers hope for translating these research findings into novel treatments. Because it appears that TMS at different frequencies has divergent effects on brain activity, combining TMS with functional brain imaging will help better delineate not only the behavioral neuropsychology of various psychiatric syndromes, but also some of the pathophysiologic circuits in the brain. Regardless of its clinical role as a new therapeutic technique, the capacity of TMS as a research tool to focally alter brain activity should lead to important advances in the understanding of brain-behavior relationships.

Vagus Nerve Stimulation

Another new somatic intervention, vagus nerve stimulation, involves stimulating the vagus nerve with electrical current (for review, see George et al. 2000b). For years, scientists have been interested in the relationship between autonomic function and the limbic system and higher cortex. Numerous studies have identified extensive projections of the vagus nerve via its sensory afferent connections in the nucleus tractus solitarius (NTS) to many areas of the brain (MacLean 1990). Bailey and Bremer (1938) reported that VNS in the cat elicited synchronized activity in the cortex of the orbital gyrus. MacLean and Pribram (1949) stimulated the vagus nerve and recorded EEGs from the cortical surface of anesthetized monkeys and found inconsistent, slow waves generated from the lateral frontal cortex (MacLean 1990). Moreover, Dell and Olson (1951) found that in awake cats with high cervical spinal section, VNS evoked a slow wave response in the anterior rhinal sulcus as well as in the amygdala.

It is not surprising that direct stimulation of the cranial nerves (direct extensions of the brain out of the skull) would interest biological psychiatrists and might have observable central effects with potential research and clinical applications in neuropsychiatry. Zabara (1985a, 1985b) first demonstrated the anticonvulsant action of VNS on experimental seizures in dogs. Although the vagus is an autonomic nerve, Zabara hypothesized that VNS could prevent or control epilepsy. On the basis of known neuroanatomy, Zabara reasoned that VNS could potentially affect areas of brain epileptic activity.

VNS refers to several different techniques used to stimulate the vagus nerve, including techniques used in animal studies in which the vagus nerve was accessed through the abdomen and diaphragm. For practically all studies in humans, VNS refers to stimulation of the left cervical vagus nerve using a commercially available device manufactured by Cyberonics, called the Neuro-Cybernetic Prosthesis (NCP) System (Schachter and Saper 1998). VNS delivered by this system has been available for treatment of refractory, partial-onset epileptic seizures in Europe since June 1994 and in the United States since July 1997. About 10,000 people worldwide, representing more than 6,500 patient-years of experience, have had this device implanted. Typically, epilepsy patients considered for VNS have had unsatisfactory seizure control with several medications and are considering VNS prior to brain surgery.

VNS is delivered through the NCP system's pulse generator—an implantable, multiprogrammable, bipolar pulse generator (the size of a pocket watch) that is implanted in the left chest wall to deliver electrical signals to the left vagus nerve through a bipolar lead. This bipolar lead is wrapped around the left vagus nerve through a separate incision at surgery and is connected to the generator through a wire that runs under the skin. The system's programming wand and programming software—along with a personal computer—provides telemetric communication with the pulse generator, which enables noninvasive programming, functional assessments (device diagnostics and interrogation), and data retrieval.

Traditionally, the vagus nerve has been considered a parasympathetic efferent nerve, which controls and regulates autonomic functions such as heart rate and gastric tone. However, the vagus (cranial nerve 10) is actually a mixed nerve composed of about 80% sensory (afferent) fibers that carry information to the brain from the head, neck, thorax, and abdomen (Foley and DuBois 1937). Interestingly, there have been very few cardiac effects of left cervical VNS, perhaps because the stimulating electrode is below the cardiac branch of the vagus nerve.

The sensory afferent cell bodies of the vagus nerve reside in the nodose ganglion and relay information to the NTS. These fibers are different from those that go to the other motor nuclei of the vagus nerve. The NTS relays this incoming sensory information to the rest of the brain through three main pathways: 1) an autonomic feedback loop, 2) direct projections to the reticular formation in the medulla, and 3) ascending projections to the forebrain largely through the parabrachial nucleus and the locus coeruleus. The parabrachial nucleus is adjacent to the locus coeruleus (one of the primary norepinephrine-containing areas of the brain) (Figure 5–3). In fact, lesioning the locus coeruleus in rats eliminates the ability of VNS to suppress seizures (Krahl et al. 1998), which shows how important this connection is for the antiepileptic effects of VNS.

The parabrachial nucleus and locus coeruleus send direct connections to every level of the forebrain, including the hypothalamus and several thalamic regions that control the insula, orbitofrontal, and prefrontal cortex. Perhaps important for mood regulation, the parabrachial nucleus and locus coeruleus have

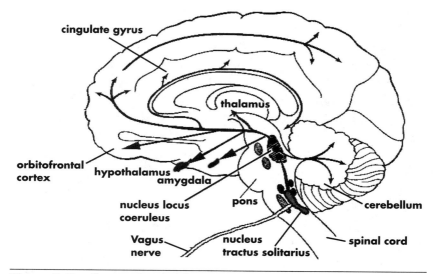

Figure 5–3. Connections of the general sensory afferent projections of the vagus nerve.

Note. Information travels from the vagus nerve to the nucleus tractus solitarius (NTS), then to the locus coeruleus. From there, information travels to limbic and higher cortical regions.

direct connections to the amygdala and the bed nucleus of the stria terminalis—structures that are very important in emotion recognition and mood regulation. For reviews of the functional neuroanatomy of depression, see George et al. (1997a) and Ketter et al. (1997).

The importance of these brainstem and limbic neuroanatomic connections is more than theoretical. The oncogene *c-fos* is a general marker for cellular activity. Studies of *c-fos* in rats during VNS revealed increased activity in the amygdala, cingulate, locus coeruleus, and hypothalamus (Naritoku et al. 1995). Recent functional MRI (fMRI) studies from our group also demonstrate how VNS alters activity in these regions.

Walker et al. (1999) outlined the key role of the NTS in VNS reduction of seizures, by microinjecting the NTS with either GABA or glutamate antagonists. An increase in GABA or a decrease in glutamate in the NTS blocked seizures. These findings suggest that VNS causes direct changes in GABA and glutamate in the NTS, with secondary changes in the function of specific limbic structures noted previously (e.g., amygdala, cingulate, insula, hippocampus).

In sum, incoming sensory (afferent) connections of the left vagus nerve provide direct projections to many of the brain regions implicated in neuropsychiatric disorders. These connections reveal how VNS might be a portal into the brainstem and connected regions. These neuroanatomic circuits likely account for many of the observed neuropsychiatric effects of VNS, and they invite additional theoretical considerations for potential research and clinical applications of VNS.

For Treatment of Epilepsy

In two double-blind studies conducted by Ben-Menachem et al. (1994) and Handforth et al. (1998), 313 patients who completed treatment had treatment-resistant epilepsy. In this difficult-to-treat group, the overall mean decline of seizure frequency was 25%–30% compared with baseline. Data from uncontrolled observations suggest that seizure control is maintained or may improve over time (Salinsky et al. 1996). Although VNS was initially controversial among neurologists, a reassessment by the American Academy of Neurology concluded that VNS is both effective and safe for the treatment of epilepsy (Fisher and Handforth 1999).

VNS delivered by the NCP system appears to be both safe and generally well tolerated. In fact, in clinical studies of epilepsy, the efferent peripheral effects of VNS to the left vagus nerve have been minimal, without significant gastrointestinal or cardiac side effects (Ben-Menachem et al. 1994; Salinsky et al. 1996). The NCP system includes mechanical and electrical safety features to minimize the possibility of high-frequency stimulation, which could lead to tissue damage. In addition, each patient is given a magnet that, when held over the pulse generator, turns off stimulation. When the magnet is removed, normal programmed stimulation resumes.

For Treatment of Depression

In addition to the neuroanatomic reasoning discussed previously, several lines of evidence provided the background for studying whether VNS could be effective for the treatment of depression, culminating in the first implant of the NCP pulse generator for this indication in July 1998 at our institution. These lines of evidence included 1) clinical observations in epilepsy patients; 2) anatomical afferent connections of the left vagus nerve to the central nervous system and to structures relevant to mood regulation; 3) the anticonvulsant activity of VNS in the context of the role of anticonvulsants or ECT (also an anticonvulsant) in treating mood disorders; 4) neurochemical studies indicating VNS effects on key neurotransmitters involved in mood regulation; and 5) evidence that VNS changes the metabolic activity of key limbic system structures.

In an initial open trial conducted at four sites by Rush et al. (2000), patients with treatment-resistant major depression were treated by adding VNS to a stable baseline of antidepressant medications. No stimulation was given for the first 2 weeks following implantation of the NCP pulse generator, creating a single-blind placebo phase and allowing for surgical recovery. All patients met eligibility criteria by not responding to at least two adequate treatment trials during the current major depressive episode (MDE) according to the Antidepressant Treatment History Form (ATHF) (Prudic et al. 1990; Sackeim et al. 1990). A total of 38 patients were enrolled in the first part of the study, 30 of whom received implants. Data are available on the 30 patients who received implantations, all of whom completed the acute treatment phase of the study, and on the post–acute phase outcomes (6-month follow-up). Seventy percent of patients had nonpsychotic, nonatypical major depressive disorder (MDD) (nearly 50% of these patients had recurrent MDD). The other 30% had bipolar disorder, depressed phase, nonrapid cycling, nonpsychotic, and nonatypical. The mean length of the current MDE was 10.3 years (SD = 12.5; range = 0.3–49.5). The median length of the current MDE was 4.3 years.

Nearly two-thirds (63%) of patients in this study had been experiencing the current MDE for 2 years or more. These were severely ill patients, and during their lifetimes, they averaged 18.4 (SD = 7.3; range = 6–39) antidepressant and mood disorder treatments, of which 9.6 (SD = 3.5; range = 3–17) were antidepressant medication trials. These patients had experienced prolonged, severe, and disabling depressive episodes and were experiencing current disabling MDEs. Thirty percent had not responded to two treatments, 7% had not responded to three, 20% had not responded to four, and 43% had not responded to 5 or more well-documented treatments that met ATHF criteria during the current major depressive episode. During the acute treatment phase of the study, patients received an average of 3.5 (SD = 1.7; median = 4; range = 0–8) other mood disorder treatments during VNS. All 30 patients had the stimulation parameters set at 500 µsec (0.5 ms) pulse width and 20 Hz ($N = 25$) or 30 Hz ($N = 5$) frequency for 30 seconds "on" and 5 minutes "off" (24 hours a day), except for 1 patient who received 250 µsec pulse width and 3 patients who received stimulation for 30 seconds "on" and 3 minutes "off." Output current ranged from 0.25 mA to 3.0 mA, depending on patient tolerance (median = 0.75 mA). Once the stimulation parameters were set at the end of a 2-week stimulation adjustment period, no patient required stimulation parameter adjustments during the acute treatment phase.

Figure 5–4 presents the $HRSD_{28}$ total scores at exit visit for each of the 30 patients and the reduction in the average (2 visits) baseline $HRSD_{28}$ in relation to the diagnosis for each patient. Overall, there was a 40% response rate using a 50% or greater reduction in baseline $HRSD_{28}$ total score to define response.

No patient had significant HRSD score changes or responded (greater than 50% depression improvement from baseline) during the first 2 weeks when the pulse generator was off. Response time appeared gradual, and early effects were suggested for patients who responded to treatment when analyzed separately ($n = 12$) (i.e., during VNS dose adjustment). However, more than half of the total reduction in response time, from HRSD score 39.1 (average at baseline) to 11.5 (average at exit), for patients who responded to treatment occurred during 6 of the 8 weeks of treatment with fixed-dose VNS. At 1-year follow-up, 91% of patients who did not respond during the acute treatment phase of the study continued to show response, and 18% of patients who did not respond during the acute treatment phase had responded. The response rate was 55% at 6 months, 52% at 9 months, and

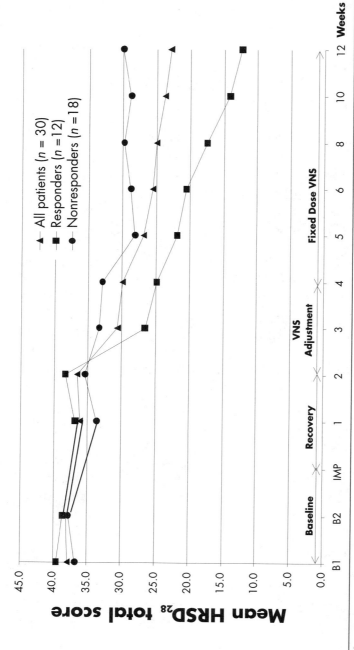

Figure 5–4. Hamilton Rating Scale for Depression (HRSD) scores for patients with treatment-resistant depression after vagus nerve stimulation (VNS).

Note. Entry HRSD scores were high, even though the patients were taking medication. In a subgroup of these patients, significant declines in HRSD scores occurred several weeks following VNS. IMP = implantation.

Source. Data from Rush et al. 2000.

46% at 1 year. An additional 11% partially responded to treatment, with 40%–49% improvement compared with baseline. Remission rates were 17% at the end of the acute treatment phase, 31% at 6 months, 33% at 9 months, and 29% at 1 year. Because VNS involves a surgical implant and is relatively expensive, it would be desirable to predict prior to surgery which patients will respond.

The only potentially significant factor during this study concerned ECT response. Only 1 of 7 patients who did not respond at all (either partially or transiently) to ECT treatment responded to VNS. The odds ratio was highest when patients who had not responded to ECT during the acute treatment phase of the study were compared with all other patients (i.e., patients who never had ECT and those who had a transient or partial ECT response). However, this relationship did not reach statistical significance ($P = 0.14$). There was also an impression that patients who received more exhaustive and aggressive pharmacotherapy during the index episode were less likely to respond. An extension of this pilot study involving 30 additional patients (all at the same initial four study sites) also indicated that the more trials a patient experienced in which he or she did not respond to various depression treatments, the more likely it was that the patient would not respond to VNS treatment. The response rate was 20%, but the depression experienced by the second group of 30 patients was significantly more treatment resistant than the depression experienced by the first group of 30.

This small extension study also indicated that patients who received VNS at lower currents had a better response rate. This paradoxical trend, which needs further investigation, may be either causal or a consequence of more severely depressed patients being treated with higher currents.

All but one patient in the initial study have elected to keep the pulse generator implanted, suggesting good tolerability. Interestingly, the first patient who received implantation (who had BPAD type 1–depressed phase) developed dysphoric hypomania, which subsided when stimulation output current was reduced. Two other cases of hypomania were seen in the ongoing follow-up extension study with an additional 30 patients (M. George and H. A.

Sackeim, personal communication, August 2000). Four serious adverse events occurred during the initial study: 1) infection, 2) leg pain, 3) agitation and panic, and 4) agitation, irritability, and dysphoria. Three patients (10%) reported abnormal wound healing, which involved a longer time for implant incisions to heal. All patients' wounds healed without significant intervention. All these events occurred at one site, and the surgeon has since modified his incision closure technique. One additional patient (3%) had a wound infection that required hospitalization and intravenous antibiotics. In the extension study, a few patients required hospitalization as a result of worsening depressive symptomatology (A. J. Rush and H. A. Sackeim, personal communication).

Given the initial study's small sample size and open design, these findings in a treatment-resistant group are preliminary. Without a randomized, sham control group, no definite conclusions can be drawn about the effectiveness of VNS for treating depression in this patient population. A multisite randomized study has begun. The severe, chronic, recurrent, and treatment-resistant nature of the depressive episodes in this patient sample suggests that only 5%–10% would be expected to improve spontaneously during the 3 months following implantation. The response rate after implantation (i.e., 40% during the acute treatment phase, 57% at 6 months) substantially exceeded these expectations. Most patients who responded to treatment sustained their improvements from the acute treatment phase in longer term follow-up, suggesting that VNS provides ongoing benefits for those who respond to treatment.

Relapse rates of 30%–60% have been commonly reported in patients with far less severe, nonresistant major depression while participating in continuation or maintenance medication treatment studies. Following ECT, relapse rates are especially high among patients with medication-resistant conditions.

Several additional points further confirm that placebo effects did not account for many of the results from the initial study. First, no patient responded in the 2-week, postimplantation, single-blind, recovery period. Additionally, follow-up data suggest that patients who initially improved retained that improvement after exiting the acute phase of the study. A pattern of sustained benefit is unlikely to reflect placebo response. These pilot results need to be replicated in a masked study before they can be accepted.

For Treatment of Other Disorders

Studies have established that VNS is an effective anticonvulsant. In addition, VNS may have antidepressant and mood-stabilizing properties. The vagus nerve is an important route of information into the central nervous system. Several theories of anxiety disorders posit that these disorders are the result of a faulty interpretation of or erratic availability of peripheral information in the central nervous system. One might suggest that altering the flow of this information could have potential in the treatment of anxiety disorders (e.g., generalized anxiety disorder, panic disorder) or irritable bowel syndrome.

Similarly, the vagus nerve contains information about hunger and satiety, as well as pain fibers. Therefore, studies on the efficacy of using VNS to treat treatment-resistant obesity, addiction, and pain are justified. Moreover, the NTS sends fibers into the dorsal raphe and areas that control levels of alertness. Thus, VNS might be considered a potential treatment for disorders of sleep and alertness such as coma and narcolepsy. In a study of 10 epilepsy patients, Kozel et al. (2000) found that high-intensity, high-frequency VNS reduced the total time patients spent in rapid eye movement (REM) sleep. In addition, REM sleep was less fragmented. Because of the known neuroanatomy of vagus nerve connections into the brain, there is reason to hope that VNS might be useful for treating other disorders and will advance our understanding about the pathophysiology of these disorders.

A study by Clark et al. (1999) hinted at the potential for using VNS to investigate brain circuits involved in memory, learning, and alertness. The authors examined word-recognition memory in 10 patients enrolled in a clinical study of VNS for the treatment of epilepsy. VNS administered after learning, during memory consolidation, caused intensity-dependent enhancement of word-recognition relative to sham stimulation. Other studies by these authors and others have shown that vagotomy attenuates the memory-enhancing properties of amphetamine, suggesting that amphetamine and other stimulants modulate emotional memory through messages about autonomic states to the brain through the vagus nerve.

Safety Issues and Side Effects

Specific VNS parameters can affect learning and memory in a classic inverted U-shape, much like peripheral stress does. This indicates that one of the mechanisms by which stress changes memory function is vagally mediated and that VNS can mimic mild peripheral stress. Better understanding of how VNS affects the brain could make VNS a powerful intervention, especially if VNS methods become less invasive. It is also likely that different VNS settings (e.g., intensity, frequency, duty cycle) have different regional effects. This implies that finding the VNS settings that maximally affect specific brain regions would be instrumental in dosing and guiding clinical trials of VNS for different neuropsychiatric conditions.

At our institution, we have succeeded in performing BOLD (blood oxygen level dependent) fMRI studies in depressed patients who received VNS pulse generator implants. Figure 5–5 shows that VNS activated many anterior paralimbic regions in these patients. Combining VNS with functional imaging offers the promise that we will better understand the neurobiology of VNS as a function of the device settings. It may also be used to individually dose VNS patients.

Deep Brain Stimulation

The most anatomically discrete, and most invasive, method of stimulating deep brain structures is *deep brain stimulation.* In this technique, a thin electrode about the width of a human hair is inserted directly into the brain. Different currents are applied at varying depths until the desired effects are found. High-frequency (> 80 Hz) electrical stimulation of the middle thalamus or subthalamic nucleus (STN) has been found effective in treating Parkinson's disease (Damier 1998; Limousin et al. 1998). Stimulation can be performed at high frequencies (> 50 Hz), which are thought to create a transient functional lesion and inhibit a brain region from normal participation in brain activity. Alternatively, low-frequency DBS may intermittently activate a region. Thus, high-frequency DBS effects on emotions and tremor are likely the result of a "functional ablation" or the switching off and inhibition of ongoing neuronal activity, although this is not well understood (Bear 1999).

For Treatment of Depression

Although DBS has not been used to treat major depression, it has been reported to affect mood. In one patient with Parkinson's disease who had never had depression before, testing of the stimulation caused the acute onset of tearfulness, sadness, and despair. These symptoms remitted immediately when the surgeon moved the stimulator away from the substantia nigra, directly below the STN (Bejjani et al. 1999). Transient acute depression was evoked 5 seconds after 130-Hz DBS of the left substantia nigra and ceased 90 seconds after DBS was stopped (Bejjani et al. 1999). Kumar et al. (1999) and Linden (1999) found that unilateral or bilateral DBS of the STN in two patients resulted in involuntary laughter and triggered imaginative associations and feelings of well-being that lasted several minutes until stimulation intensity was lowered or DBS was discontinued. This emotional reaction was accompanied by improvement in parkinsonian symptoms and led Linden (1999) to conclude that "the STN is part of a neuronal network that may influence the emotional state and cause laughter—or depression." Our institution has an ongoing National Institutes of Health–funded project that is building on these observations by using interleaved TMS/fMRI to define the neuronal network associated with the STN and mood effects and to determine if stimulation of this network has potential in treating depression in Parkinson's disease.

Early studies of diagnostic DBS prior to neurosurgical ablations also demonstrated emotional reactions. Much of this work involved stimulation of the thalamus. For example, microstimulation of the nucleus ventralis caudalis (somatosensory) was accompanied by a strong affective component of visceral pain

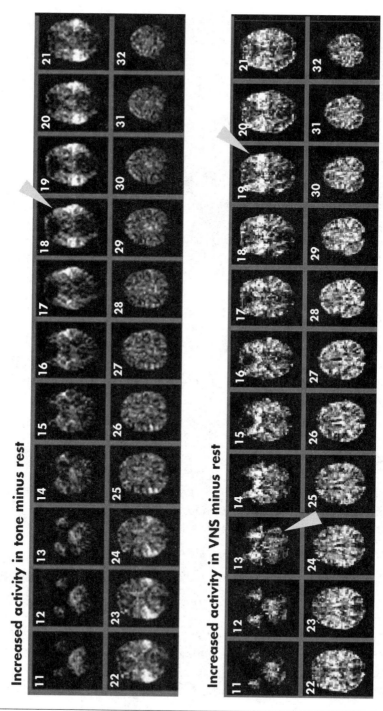

Increased activity in tone minus rest

Increased activity in VNS minus rest

Figure 5–5. Statistical parametric maps of regional brain activity in four depressed patients during vagus nerve stimulation (VNS).

Note. The gray scales show areas of significantly increased activity compared with rest when patients listened to a tone (top) and when the VNS device was on for 7 seconds (bottom). Brighter areas are more significantly active. The images are numbered from the bottom of the brain (11) to the top (32). Note the increased signal as expected in the auditory cortex when patients heard the tone (arrow). In contrast, VNS caused increased blood flow in many brain regions, particularly in the medial temporal lobes, orbitofrontal cortex, insula, and prefrontal cortex. (Pooled data from four subjects [DO1]; average 6 months post-acute phase, 7 seconds VNS on, 108 seconds VNS off, VNS 0.25–0.75 mA, 20 Hz, 500 μsec *p* width.)

Source. Daryl Bohning, Ph.D., Center for Advanced Imaging Research, Medical University of South Carolina, Charleston, South Carolina.

similar to that previously observed in a patient during a panic attack (Lenz et al. 1995). Weeping, anxiety, and depression were reported to be elicited during neurosurgery in unanesthetized patients with Parkinson's disease with 32 Hz of stimulation for several seconds of thalamic nuclei as well as from pallidum, septum, and hypothalamus. Different emotional reactions occurred when the nucleus ventralis lateralis was stimulated with a floating electrode (Illinski 1970). Summarizing the effects of diagnostic and therapeutic DBS via long-term implanted electrodes in a large sample of patients with Parkinson's disease, Smirnov (1976) indicated that positive emotional states occurred after stimulation of the centrum medianum area of the thalamus. Interestingly, high-frequency (ablative) DBS as well as stereotaxic destruction of the anterior thalamic nuclei resulted in relief from intractable agitated depression (Mark et al. 1970). And finally, the thalamus was one of the brain structures in which Heath and colleagues recorded EEG correlates of pleasure during orgasm (Heath 1972).

Safety Issues and Side Effects

Before clinicians can use DBS to treat primary mood disorders, more studies of the mood effects of DBS in patients with Parkinson's disease and obsessive-compulsive disorder are needed. Because of its invasiveness, DBS will likely be used only for patients who have not responded to less invasive techniques, including the other MIBS techniques such as TMS, VNS, and ECT/MST.

Conclusion

Knowledge of the regional neuroanatomic deficits of depression is rapidly catching up with the pharmacological expertise of modern psychiatry. This knowledge is serving as the background for a renaissance of several new somatic interventions that will change the way clinicians think about and treat depression. As our knowledge expands, we must begin to assess whether these new interventions, alone or in combination with other treatments, will be effective in preventing recurrences of major depression.

References

Avery DH, Claypoole K, Robinson L, et al: Repetitive transcranial magnetic stimulation in the treatment of medication-resistant depression: preliminary data. J Nerv Ment Dis 187:114–117, 1999

BaileyP, Bremer F: A sensory cortical representation of the vagus nerve. J Neurophysiol 1:405–412, 1938

Barker AT, Jalinous R, Freeston IL: Non-invasive magnetic stimulation of the human motor cortex. Lancet 1:1106–1107, 1985

Bear MF: Homosynaptic long-term depression: a mechanism for memory? Proc Natl Acad Sci U S A 96:9457–9458, 1999

Beck AT, Beamesderfer A: Assessment of depression: the depression inventory. Mod Probl Pharmacopsychiatry 7:151–169, 1974

Beer B: Uber das Auftreten einer objectiven Lichtempfindung in magnetischen Felde. Klinische Wochenzeitschrift 15:108–109, 1902

Bejjani BP, Damier P, Arnulf I, et al: Transient acute depression induced by high-frequency deep brain stimulation. N Engl J Med 340:1476–1480, 1999

Belmaker RH, Fleischmann A: Transcranial magnetic stimulation: a potential new frontier in psychiatry. Biol Psychiatry 38:419–421, 1995

Ben-Menachem E, Manon-Espaillat R, Ristanovic R, et al: Vagus nerve stimulation for treatment of partial seizures, 1: a controlled study of effect on seizures. Epilepsia 35:616–626, 1994

Berman RM, Narasimhan M, Sanacora G, et al: A randomized clinical trial of repetitive transcranial magnetic stimulation in the treatment of major depression. Biol Psychiatry 47:332–337, 2000

Bohning DE: Introduction and overview of TMS physics, in Transcranial Magnetic Stimulation in Neuropsychiatry. Edited by George MS, Belmaker RH. Washington, DC, American Psychiatric Press, 2000, pp 13–44

Breitner JCS, Husain MM, Figiel GS, et al: Cerebral white matter disease in late-onset paranoid psychosis. Biol Psychiatry 28:266–274, 1990

Bremner JD, Innis RB, Salomon RM, et al: Positron emission tomography measurement of cerebral metabolic correlates of trytophan depletion–induced depressive relapse. Arch Gen Psychiatry 54:364–374, 1997

Clark KB, Naritoku DK, Smith DC, et al: Enhanced recognition memory following vagus nerve stimulation in human subjects. Nature Neuroscience 2:94–98, 1999

Coffey CE, Figiel GS, Djang WT, et al: Leukoencephalopathy in elderly depressed patients referred for ECT. Biol Psychiatry 24:143–161, 1988

Coffey CE, Figiel GS, Djang WT, et al: White matter hyperintensity on magnetic resonance imaging: clinical and neuroanatomic correlates in the depressed elderly. J Neuropsychiatry Clin Neurosci 1:135–144, 1989

Damier P: The stimulation of deep cerebral structures in the treatment of Parkinson's disease (abstract). Eur Neuropsychopharmacol 8: S89, 1998

Dell P, Olson R: Projections 'secondaires' mesencephaliques, diencephaliques et amygdaliennes des afferences viscerales vagales. C R Soc Biol 145:1088–1091, 1951

Dolan RJ, Bench CJ, Liddle PF, et al: Dorsolateral prefrontal cortex dysfunction in the major psychoses: symptom or disease specificity? J Neurol Neurosurg Psychiatry 56:1290–1294, 1993

Drevets WC, Videen TO, Price JL, et al: A functional anatomical study of unipolar depression. J Neurosci 12:3628–3641, 1992

Ebert D, Feistel H, Barocka A: Effects of sleep deprivation on the limbic system and the frontal lobes in affective disorders: a study with Tc-99m-HMPAO SPECT. Psychiatry Res 40:247–251, 1991

Ebert D, Feistel H, Barocka A, et al: Increased limbic flow and total sleep deprivation in major depression with melancholia. Psychiatry Res 55:101–109, 1994

Epstein CM, Schwartzberg DG, Davey KR, et al: Localizing the site of magnetic brain stimulation in humans. Neurology 40:666–670, 1990

Epstein CM, Lah JJ, Meador K, et al: Optimum stimulus parameters for lateralized suppression of speech with magnetic brain stimulation. Neurology 47:1590–1593, 1996

Figiel GS, Epstein C, McDonald WM, et al: The use of rapid-rate transcranial magnetic stimulation (rTMS) in refractory depressed patients. J Neuropsychiatry Clin Neurosci 10:20–25, 1998

Fisher RS, Handforth A: Reassessment: vagus nerve stimulation for epilepsy: a report of the Therapeutics and Technology Assessment Subcommittee of the American Academy of Neurology. Neurology 53: 666–669, 1999

Foley JO, DuBois F: Quantitative studies of the vagus nerve in the cat, I: the ratio of sensory and motor studies. J Comp Neurol 67:49–67, 1937

George MS, Belmaker RH (eds): Transcranial Magnetic Stimulation in Neuropsychiatry. Washington, DC, American Psychiatric Press, 2000

George MS, Wassermann EM: Rapid-rate transcranial magnetic stimulation and ECT. Convuls Ther 10:251–254, 1994

George MS, Wassermann EM, Williams WA, et al: Daily repetitive transcranial magnetic stimulation (rTMS) improves mood in depression. NeuroReport 6:1853–1856, 1995

George MS, Post RM, Ketter TA, et al: Neural mechanisms of mood disorders. Current Review of Mood and Anxiety Disorders. 1:71–83, 1997a

George MS, Wassermann EM, Kimbrell TA, et al: Mood improvement following daily left prefrontal repetitive transcranial magnetic stimulation in patients with depression: a placebo-controlled crossover trial. Am J Psychiatry 154:1752–1756, 1997b

George MS, Lisanby SH, Sackeim HA: Transcranial magnetic stimulation: applications in neuropsychiatry. Arch Gen Psychiatry 56:300–311, 1999a

George MS, Nahas Z, Lomarev M, et al: How knowledge of regional brain dysfunction in depression will enable new somatic treatments in the next millennium. CNS Spectrums: The International Journal of Neuropsychiatric Medicine 4:53–61, 1999b

George MS, Nahas Z, Molloy M, et al: A controlled trial of daily left prefrontal cortex TMS for treating depression. Biol Psychiatry 48:962–970, 2000a

George MS, Sackeim HA, Rush AJ, et al: Vagus nerve stimulation: a new tool for brain research and therapy. Biol Psychiatry 47:287–295, 2000b

George R, Salinsky M, Kuzniecky R, et al: Vagus nerve stimulation for treatment of partial seizures: 2. Long-term follow-up on first 67 patients exiting a controlled study. Epilepsia 35:637–643, 1994

Greenberg BD, George MS, Dearing J, et al: Effect of prefrontal repetitive transcranial magnetic stimulation (rTMS) in obsessive-compulsive disorder: a preliminary study. Am J Psychiatry 154:867–869, 1997

Greenberg BD, Ziemann U, Harmon A, et al: Reduced intracortical inhibition in obsessive-compulsive disorder on transcranial magnetic stimulation. Lancet 352:881–882, 1998

Grisaru N, Yarovslavsky U, Abarbanel J, et al: Transcranial magnetic stimulation in depression and schizophrenia. Eur Neuropsychopharmacol 4:287–288, 1994

Grisaru N, Chudakov B, Yaroslavsky Y, et al: Transcranial magnetic stimulation in mania: a controlled study. Am J Psychiatry 155:1608–1610, 1998

Grunhaus L, Dannon P, Schrieber S: Effects of transcranial magnetic stimulation on severe depression: similarities with ECT (abstract). Biol Psychiatry 43(76s):254, 1998

Grunhaus L, Dannon PN, Screiber S, et al: Repetitive transcranial magnetic stimulation is as effective as electroconvulsive therapy in the treatment of nondelusional major depressive disorder: an open study. Biol Psychiatry 47:314–324, 2000

Handforth A, DeGiorgio CM, Schachter SC, et al: Vagus nerve stimulation therapy for partial-onset seizures: a randomized active-control trial. Neurology 51:48–55, 1998

Heath RG: Pleasure and brain activity in man. Deep and surface electroencephalograms during orgasm. J Nerv Ment Dis 154:3–18, 1972

Hoffman R, Boutros N, Berman R, et al: Transcranial magnetic stimulation and hallucinated "voices" (abstract). Biol Psychiatry 43(93s):310, 1998

Hoflich G, Kasper S, Hufnagel A, et al: Application of transcranial magnetic stimulation in treatment of drug-resistant major depression—a report of two cases. Human Psychopharmacology 8:361–365, 1993

Homberg V, Stephan KM, Netz J: Transcranial stimulation of motor cortex in upper motor neurone syndrome: its relation to the motor deficit. Electroencephalogr Clin Neurophysiol 81:377–388, 1991

Illinski IA: Emotional-affective reactions evoked by electrostimulation of the ventrolateral nucleus of the optic thalamus. Vopr Neirokhir 34(4):26–29, 1970

Impastato DJ: The story of electroshock treatment. Am J Psychiatry 116:1113–1114, 1960

Ketter TA, George MS, Kimbrell TA, et al: Functional brain imaging in mood and anxiety disorders. Current Review of Mood and Anxiety Disorders 1:96–112, 1997

Kimbrell TA, Little JT, Dunn RT, et al: Frequency dependence of antidepressant response to left prefrontal repetitive transcranial magnetic stimulation (rTMS) as a function of baseline cerebral glucose metabolism. Biol Psychiatry 46:1603–1613, 1999

Klein E, Kreinin I, Chistyakov A, et al: Therapeutic efficacy of right prefrontal slow repetitive transcranial magnetic stimulation in major depression: a double-blind controlled study. Arch Gen Psychiatry 56:315–320, 1999

Kolbinger HM, Hoflich G, Hufnagel A, et al: Transcranial magnetic stimulation (TMS) in the treatment of major depression—a pilot study. Human Psychopharmacology 10:305–310, 1995

Kozel FA, Nahas Z, DeBrux C, et al: How the distance from coil to cortex relates to age, motor threshold and possibly the antidepressant response to repetitive transcranial magnetic stimulation. J Neuropsychiatry Clin Neurosci 12:376–384, 2000

Krahl SE, Clark KB, Smith DC, et al: Locus coeruleus lesions suppress the seizure attenuating effects of vagus nerve stimulation. Epilepsia 39:709–714, 1998

Kumar R, Lozano AM, Sime E, et al: Comparative effects of unilateral and bilateral subthalamic nucleus deep brain stimulation. Neurology 53:561–566, 1999

Lenz FA, Gracely RH, Romanoski AJ, et al: Stimulation in the human somatosensory thalamus can reproduce both the affective and sensory dimensions of previously experienced pain. National Medicine 1:910–913, 1995

Limousin P, Krack P, Pollak P, et al: Electrical stimulation of the subthalamic nucleus in advanced Parkinson's disease. N Engl J Med 339: 1105–1111, 1998

Linden DJ: The return of the spike: postsynaptic action potentials an the induction of LTP and LTD. Neuron 22:661–666, 1999

Lisanby SH, Sackeim HA: Therapeutic brain interventions and the nature of emotion, in The Neuropsychology of Emotion. Edited by Borod J. New York, Oxford University Press, 2000

Lisanby SH, Luber B, Finck D, et al: Primate models of transcranial magnetic stimulation (abstract). Biol Psychiatry 41(76s), 1998a

Lisanby SH, Luber B, Schroeder C, et al: Intracerebral measurement of rTMS and ECS induced voltage in vivo. Biol Psychiatry 43:100s, 1998b

Lisanby SH, Luber BM, Finck D, et al: Magnetic stimulation therapy: a novel convulsive technique (abstract). Biol Psychiatry (in press)

Little JT, Kimbrell TA, Wassermann EM, et al: Lack of cognitive side effects of 1 and 20 Hz repetitive transcranial magnetic stimulation in depression. Neuropsychiatry Neuropsychol Behav Neurol 1999 (in press)

Loo C, Mitchell P, Sachdev P, et al: rTMS: a sham-controlled trial in medication-resistant depression (abstract). Biol Psychiatry 43(95s):317, 1998

Loo CK, Taylor JL, Gandevia SC, et al: Transcranial magnetic stimulation (TMS) in controlled treatment studies: are some "sham" forms active? Biol Psychiatry 47:325–331, 2000

Lorberbaum JP, Wassermann EM: Safety concerns of transcranial magnetic stimulation, in Transcranial Magnetic Stimulation in Neuropsychiatry. Edited by George MS, Belmaker RH. Washington, DC, American Psychiatric Press, 2000, pp 141–162

MacLean PD: The Triune Brain in Evolution: Role in Paleocerebral Functions. New York, Plenum, 1990

Marangell LB, George MS, Callahan AM, et al: Effects of intrathecal thyrotropin-releasing hormone (protirelin) in refractory depressed patients. Arch Gen Psychiatry 54:214–222, 1997

Mark VH, Barry H, McLardy T, et al: The destruction of both anterior thalamic nuclei in a patient with intractable agitated depression. J Nerv Ment Dis 150:266–272, 1970

Mayberg HS, Brannan SK, Mahurin RK, et al: Cingulate function in depression: a potential predictor of treatment response. NeuroReport 8:1057–1061, 1997

Mirsky AF, Anthony BJ, Duncan CC, et al: Analysis of the elements of attention: a neuropsychological approach. Neuropsychol Rev 2:109–145, 1991

Nahas Z, George MS, Lorberbaum JP, et al: SPECT and PET in neuropsychiatry. Primary Psychiatry 5:52–59, 1998

Nahas Z, McConnell K, Collins S, et al: Could left prefrontal rTMS modify negative symptoms and attention in schizophrenia? (abstract). Biol Psychiatry 45(37S):120, 1999a

Nahas Z, Teneback CT, Speer AM, et al: The effect of frequency and distance of TMS on prefrontal cortex blood flow (abstract). Human Brain Mapping 9:236, 1999b

Nahas Z, DeBrux C, Chandler V, et al: Lack of significant changes on magnetic resonance scans before and after 2 weeks of daily left prefrontal repetitive transcranial magnetic stimulation for depression. J ECT 16:380–390, 2000

Naritoku DK, Terry WJ, Helfert RH: Regional induction of fos immunoreactivity in the brain by anticonvulsant stimulation of the vagus nerve. Epilepsy Res 22:53–62, 1995

Nobler MS, Sackeim HA, Prohovnik I, et al: Regional cerebral blood flow in mood disorders, III. Treatment and clinical response. Arch Gen Psychiatry 51:884–897, 1994

Nobler MS, Teneback CC, Nahas Z, et al: Structural and functional neuroimaging of ECT and TMS. Depression and Anxiety 12:144–156, 2000

Pascual-Leone A, Grafman J, Hallett M: Modulation of cortical motor output maps during development of implicit and explicit knowledge. Science 263:1287–1289, 1994a

Pascual-Leone A, Valls-Sole J, Brasil-Neto JP, et al: Akinesia in Parkinson's disease. I. Shortening of simple reaction times with focal, single-pulse transcranial magnetic stimulation. Neurology 44:884–891, 1994b

Pascual-Leone A, Valls-Sole J, Brasil-Neto JP, et al: Akinesia in Parkinson's disease. II. Effects of subthreshold repetitive transcranial motor cortex stimulation. Neurology 44:892–898, 1994c

Pascual-Leone A, Valls-Sole J, Wasserman EM, et al: Responses to rapid-rate transcranial magnetic stimulation of the human motor cortex. Brain 117:847–858, 1994d

Pascual-Leone A, Catala MD, Pascual AP: Lateralized effect of rapid-rate transcranial magnetic stimulation of the prefrontal cortex on mood. Neurology 46:499–502, 1996a

Pascual-Leone A, Rubio B, Pallardo F, et al: Beneficial effect of rapid-rate transcranial magnetic stimulation of the left dorsolateral prefrontal cortex in drug-resistant depression. Lancet 348:233–237, 1996b

Prudic J, Sackeim HA, Devanand DP: Medication resistance and clinical response to electroconvulsive therapy. Psychiatry Res 31:287–296, 1990

Reutens DC, Berkovic SF, MacDonell RA, et al: Magnetic stimulation of the brain in generalized epilepsy: reversal of cortical hyperexcitability by anticonvulsants. Ann Neurol 34:351–355, 1993a

Reutens DC, Puce A, Berkovic SF: Cortical hyperexcitability in progressive myoclonus epilepsy: a study with transcranial magnetic stimulation. Neurology 43:186–192, 1993b

Rush AJ, George MS, Sackeim HA, et al: Vagus nerve stimulation (VNS) for treatment-resistant depressions: a multicenter study. Biol Psychiatry 47:276–286, 2000

Sackeim HA, Prudic J, Devanand DP, et al: The impact of medication resistance and continuation pharmacotherapy on relapse following response to electroconvulsive therapy in major depression. J Clin Psychopharmacol 10:96–104, 1990

Sackeim HA, Prudic J, Devanand DP, et al: Effects of stimulus intensity and electrode placement on the efficacy and cognitive effects of electroconvulsive therapy. N Engl J Med 328:839–846, 1993

Sackeim HA, Prudic J, Devanand DP, et al: A prospective, randomized, double-blind comparison of bilateral and right unilateral electroconvulsive therapy at different stimulus intensities. Arch Gen Psychiatry 57:425–434, 2000

Salinsky MC, Uthman BM, Ristanovic RK, et al: Vagus nerve stimulation for the treatment of medically intractable seizures: results of a 1-year open-extension trial. Arch Neurol 53:1176–1180, 1996

Schachter SC, Saper CB: Vagus nerve stimulation. Epilepsia 39:677–686, 1998

Teneback CC, Nahas Z, Speer AM, et al: Changes in prefrontal cortex and paralimbic activity in depression following two weeks of daily left prefrontal TMS. J Neuropsychiatry Clin Neurosci 11:426–435, 1999

Triggs WJ, McCoy KJ, Greer R, et al: Effects of left frontal transcranial magnetic stimulation on depressed mood, cognition, and corticomotor threshold. Biol Psychiatry 45:1440–1446, 1999

Walker BR, Easton A, Gale K: Regulation of limbic motor seizures by GABA and glutamate transmission in nucleus tractus solitarius. Epilepsia 40:1051–1057, 1999

Wassermann EM: Risk and safety of repetitive transcranial magnetic stimulation: report and suggested guidelines from the International Workshop on the Safety of Repetitive Transcranial Magnetic Stimulation, June 5–7, 1996. Electroencephalogr Clin Neurophysiol 108:1–16, 1998

Wassermann EM, McShane LM, Hallett M, et al: Noninvasive mapping of muscle representations in human motor cortex. Electroencephalogr Clin Neurophysiol 85:1–8, 1992

Wassermann EM, Wedegaertner FR, Ziemann U, et al: Crossed reduction of motor cortex excitability by 1 Hz transcranial magnetic stimulation. Neurosci Lett 250:141–144, 1998

Wu JC, Gillin JC, Buchsbaum MS, et al: Effect of sleep deprivation on brain metabolism of depressed patients. Am J Psychiatry 149:538–543, 1992

Zabara J: Peripheral control of hypersynchronous discharge in epilepsy. Electroencephalogr Clin Neurophysiol 61(suppl):S162, 1985a

Zabara J: Time course of seizure control to brief, repetitive stimuli (abstract). Epilepsia 26:518, 1985b

Ziemann U, Hallett M: Basic neurophysiological studies with TMS, in Transcranial Magnetic Stimulation in Neuropsychiatry. Edited by George MS, Belmaker RH. Washington, DC, American Psychiatric Press, 2000, pp. 45–98

Chapter 6

Clinical Prevention of Recurrent Depression

The Need for Paradigm Shifts

John F. Greden, M.D.

As emphasized in traditional publications (Angst et al. 1973; Zis and Goodwin 1979a), major textbook reviews (Goodwin and Jamison 1990), and Chapters 1, 3, and 4 in this volume, powerful evidence reveals that major depressive disorder (MDD) is an episodic, recurrent disorder that induces a profound burden—a burden that grows steadily with each new episode. The challenge of preventing recurrences of MDD is arguably among the most important in medicine. A compilation of steps to accomplish this would be valuable for clinicians and families; this chapter presents these steps.

Knowledge heals. Our knowledge about recurrent depression is rapidly accumulating, and there comes a time when clinicians interested in applying evidence-based medicine must respond to the preponderance of evidence. Have we attained enough evidence to guide us in the treatment of recurrent depression? The answer appears to be strongly affirmative. It is time to prioritize prevention of MDD recurrences. It is time to use our knowledge. It is time for major paradigm shifts.

MDD Versus Other Diseases: What Can We Learn?

Before reviewing studies on depression recurrences, we might ask whether we can learn anything by comparing MDD with other chronic biologic diseases for which stopping progression remains a challenge, but where advances have been made (see Table 6–1). What have clinicians in other fields learned?

Clinical symptoms on which diagnoses are based are generally preceded by less specific and less severe prodromal symptoms. Often such milder symptoms are not detected. Most chronic diseases (e.g., diabetes, heart disease, schizophrenia, bipolar disorder) are characterized by lifetime progression unless actively treated. This is also true for MDD.

Continuing the comparison of MDD with diabetes and heart disease, the earlier the intervention, the better the outcome (Frasure-Smith and Lesperance 2000; Frasure-Smith et al. 2000). Indeed, the American College of Cardiology refined its diagnostic definition of myocardial infarction in order to encourage earlier intervention (Roan 2000). The same shift is occurring for schizophrenia. Lieberman and Fenton (2000) pointed out that "the first episode of schizophrenia is a critical therapeutic opportunity, and if patients are treated promptly and effectively, good outcomes can be achieved" (p. 1727), a viewpoint shared by other investigators (Ho et al. 2000; McGlashan 1999). Yet, as Lieberman and Fenton also noted, "Throughout the world, individuals suffering a first episode of psychosis experience an alarming delay between the onset of psychotic symptoms and the initiation of treatment" (p. 1727). Similar delays between onset, diagnosis, and treatment have been observed for bipolar disorder (see Chapter 4 in this volume), and may be even more pronounced for those with MDD, sometimes extending to years or decades.

During such delays, for most major medical illnesses, undesirable consequences occur. Out-of-control diabetes and heart disease are associated with progressive tissue damage in various organs (Goff et al. 1999). Comparably, both recurrent chronic depression (Sheline et al. 1996) and schizophrenia (Lieberman 1999) appear to be associated with neuronal degeneration. For schizophrenia, MDD, and bipolar disorder, questions remain about whether there are any relationships between the duration of previous psychosis and changes in regional brain volumes, or whether the reported morphological changes in the brain are reversible (Starkman et al. 1999). Lacking such information, our focus should

Table 6–1. Comparison of major depressive disorder (MDD) with other chronic, progressive disorders

	Diabetes	Cardiovascular disease	Schizophrenia	Bipolar disorder	MDD
Milder, prodromal symptoms	Yes	Yes	Yes	Yes	Yes
Laboratory tests available to aid diagnosis	Yes	Yes	No	No	No
Months to years of symptom progression before diagnosis	Yes	Yes	Yes	Yes	Yes
Delayed detection and lack of treatment induce tissue damage or degeneration	Yes (multiple organs)	Yes (multiple organs)	Yes (brain)	Probably similar to unipolar disorder (not studied)	Yes (brain, heart)
Damage linked to duration	Yes	Yes	Probable	Probable	Probable
Progressive clinical deterioration if untreated	Yes	Yes	Yes	Yes	Yes
Treatment resistance	Yes	Yes	Yes	Probable	Probable
Early detection and treatment prevents clinical and tissue deterioration and treatment resistance	Yes	Yes	Probable	Probable	Probable
Treatment reverses tissue deterioration in patients with chronic and severe illness	Not known	Probable	Not known	Not known	Not known
Extended maintenance treatments available to sustain wellness	Yes	Yes	Yes	Yes	Yes
Maintenance treatments are widely recognized as essential and regularly prescribed	Yes	Yes	Yes	Yes	No
Adherence a problem when maintenance treatment prescribed	Yes	Yes	Yes	Yes	Yes

be prevention. The neurotoxic brain damage associated with untreated schizophrenia has been hypothesized to present clinically as deterioration and treatment resistance (Lieberman 1999; Lieberman and Fenton 2000; Wyatt 1991), and the same is now being inferred for recurrent chronic MDD (Sheline et al. 1996, 1998).

As an additional comparison, within the treatment domain, "tight" clinical management of diabetes is not perfect but is nevertheless effective in slowing progression and disability. Similarly, strategies to prevent recurrences of and long-term deterioration associated with MDD, although not perfect, are available and effective. Failure to use maintenance-of-wellness programs may be the major reason for the high disability measures for most of these diseases; however, for MDD, it is the norm and produces profound consequences (Murray and Lopez 1996) (see also Chapter 1 in this volume).

Changes are occurring in heart disease and diabetes prevention. Cardiovascular clinicians have begun prioritizing prevention of initial and recurrent heart attacks, emphasizing greater use of extended maintenance treatment of hypertension, prescribing antilipid and antiarrhythmic medications, encouraging stress reduction and exercise, and concomitantly treating coexisting depression. Prevention of progression similarly became a key focus for diabetes clinicians. Our growing knowledge now permits us to make prevention of progression a key focus for clinicians who treat MDD.

Clinical Strategies for Preventing Recurrences of Major Depressive Disorder

Strategies for preventing MDD recurrences have understandably focused on proven treatments for acute episodes of MDD. These include antidepressants and mood stabilizers (pharmacotherapy), electroconvulsive therapy, and various psychotherapies, notably cognitive-behavioral therapy and interpersonal therapy. Sadly, only antidepressant pharmacotherapy has an adequate database, although quality assessments of combination pharmacotherapy and psychotherapy are becoming more common (see Chapter 3 in this volume).

Studies on prevention of MDD recurrences have accumulated over the past quarter of a century. Many studies are limited by inadequate dosages, a treatment duration of only 1–2 years, failure to control for concomitant treatments, inadequate monitoring of adherence, and heterogeneous populations. Nevertheless, as reflected in Table 6–2, consistent evidence has emerged from studies that are acceptably controlled and at least 1 year in duration:

- Antidepressant and mood stabilizing medications (pharmacotherapy) perform better than placebo and no treatment in all studies, and in most studies, achieve significance.
- Antidepressant and mood stabilizing medications (pharmacotherapy) perform better than psychotherapeutic interventions, which are superior to placebo and no treatment.
- For patients with a history of multiple episodes of MDD, relapses and recurrences tend to occur early after maintenance treatment is discontinued, generally within 1 year, often sooner. (If patients and families were aware of that fact, adherence to maintenance treatment might improve.)
- Adequacy of treatments is essential, regardless of what modalities are employed.
- The small number of maintenance studies combining pharmacotherapy and psychotherapy suggest that combination treatment may be the optimal approach.
- Special steps to promote adherence with maintenance treatment are essential, even in clinical trials.
- Many practical research questions remain unanswered.

To reiterate, there comes a time when clinicians interested in applying evidence-based medicine must respond to the preponderance of evidence, even if all research questions are not fully answered. To paraphrase an axiom, absence of evidence is not evidence of absence. According to the data presented in Table 6–2, the time to respond appears to have arrived for prevention of MDD recurrences. Because new knowledge is essential for continued progress, however, closure must be avoided, and new studies must be a priority.

Table 6–2. Efficacy of antidepressant maintenance treatment versus placebo in preventing recurrences of major depressive disorder (MDD)

Study	Medication	Antidepressant	Relapse (%) Placebo	Significance
Prien et al. 1973	Imipramine	29	85	0.01
Prien et al. 1973	Lithium	41	85	0.05
Coppen et al. 1973	Amitriptyline	0	31	0.01
Prien et al. 1973	Lithium	57	71	0.05
Schou 1979	Lithium	29	84	0.001
Kane et al. 1982	Lithium	29	100	0.001
Kane et al. 1982	Imipramine	67	100	NS
Bjork 1983	Zimeldine	32	84	0.001
Glen et al. 1984	Amitriptyline	43	88	0.05
Glen et al. 1984	Lithium	42	88	0.05
Prien et al. 1984	Imipramine	44	71	0.05
Montgomery et al. 1988	Fluoxetine	26	57	0.001
Georgotas et al. 1989	Phenelzine	13	65	0.05
Frank et al. 1990	Imipramine	21	78	0.001
Rouillon et al. 1991	Maprotiline	16	32	0.01
Jakovljevic and Mewett 1991	Imipramine	12	23	0.05

Table 6–2. Efficacy of antidepressant maintenance treatment versus placebo in preventing recurrences of major depressive disorder (MDD) *(continued)*

Study	Medication	Antidepressant	Relapse (%) Placebo	Significance
Jakovljevic and Mewett 1991	Paroxetine	14	23	NS
Robinson et al. 1991	Phenelzine	10	75	0.001
Doogan and Caillard 1992	Sertraline	13	46	0.001
Montgomery and Dunbar 1993	Paroxetine	15	39	0.01
Buysse et al. 1996	Nortriptyline	27	62	0.003
Bauer et al. 2000[a]	Lithium	0	47	0.006

Note. NS = not significant.

[a] An augmenting clinical trial.

Source. Adapted with permission from Greden JF: "Antidepressant Maintenance Medications," in *Pharmacotherapy for Mood, Anxiety, and Cognitive Disorders.* Edited by Halbreich U, Montgomery S. Washington, DC, 2000, pp. 315–330. Copyright 2000, American Psychiatric Press.

Pressing Research Challenges

A few of the most important research challenges deserve comment because they are important to interpreting and improving recommendations for preventing MDD recurrences (see Table 6–3).

First, developing laboratory tests to identify patients at risk for recurrences, especially among those whose health has been compromised by recurrences, is a high priority. Such laboratory tests can be tremendously valuable in identifying patients at risk for disorders such as heart disease and diabetes. Promising laboratory tests for recurrent depression include microarray genetic assessment, serial sleep electroencephalogram (EEG) or neuroendocrine measures (Greden et al. 1983), genotyping of polymorphisms of serotonin and other transporters, serial brain imaging measures with more sensitive MRI magnets, and clinical assessment of clock gene function. Lacking such tests for now, we must resort to standardizing a cluster of clinical predictors. Because no single predictor is powerful enough, a recommended starting point for clinical research is to quantify multiple clinical and epidemiological variables already reported to be associated with higher risk of recurrent MDD and integrate them into a matrix that helps estimate the risk of recurrence. Recommended components of this list include the following:

- Number of previous episodes (Greden 1993)
- Number of days spent depressed during lifetime (Sheline et al. 1999)
- Family history of MDD (Kendler et al. 1993a, 1993b, 1999)
- History of key clinical variables, especially early age at onset (Pine et al. 1998)
- Chronic dysthymia (Keller 1999)
- Psychosis (Nierenberg and Amsterdam 1990)
- Treatment resistance (Nierenberg and Amsterdam 1990)
- Prompt relapse or recurrence following previous discontinuation of treatment (Frank et al. 1990; Kupfer et al. 1992)
- Previous suicidal behavior or persistent suicidal ideation during depressive episodes (Pfeffer 1986)
- Current severity; concurrent medical illnesses, or personal or

Table 6–3.   Research challenges for recurrent major depressive disorder (MDD)

Develop genetic screening and other laboratory tests, and use alternative methods (e.g., genetic microarray strategies, high-resolution magnetic resonance imaging [MRI] of the brain, assessment of delta sleep ratio) to identify individuals at high risk for MDD and patients at risk for recurrences of MDD.

Until predictive laboratory tests are available, develop and standardize clinical criteria to identify patients who need extended maintenance treatment.

Determine whether extended maintenance antidepressant treatment is effective in children and adolescents.

Clarify interactions among stress, gonadal hormones, and serotonin and other neurotransmitters in women, and develop treatment strategies for use during reproductive transitions.

Determine how side-effect, cost, and convenience profiles affect treatment adherence.

Determine optimal required doses of various antidepressant medications.

Determine which combination treatments work most effectively.

Compute large-sample risk-benefit ratios to compare "careful watching" with extended antidepressant treatment.

Serially monitor MRI scans of the brain and gene expression, and use other laboratory measures to determine whether and how neuronal degenerative changes progress and how they might be stopped or reversed.

Assess whether new antidepressant treatments can help prevent recurrences (e.g., vagus nerve stimulation; repetitive transcranial magnetic stimulation; combinations of sleep deprivation, pindolol, and mood stabilizers).

Determine how the recently discovered clock gene controls circadian rhythmicity, and assess whether treatment interventions can alter its functions and be used to help prevent recurrences.

Assess the benefits of nutraceuticals (e.g., St.-John's-wort), and educate patients and families about potential problems.

occupational circumstances that make any future depressive recurrence truly "hazardous"

- Presence of recurrences accompanied by one or more selected laboratory variables, notably 1) persistent abnormalities of stress hormone regulation with elevated glucocorticoids or abnormal hypothalamic-pituitary-adrenal measures (Greden et al. 1983); 2) magnetic resonance imaging (MRI) evidence of hippocampal or amygdala atrophy not attributable to other causes (Sheline et al. 1996); or 3) selected sleep EEG abnormalities (Kupfer et al. 1994; Perlis et al. 1997).

Why are these items on the list? Each has been reported to be associated with increased risk for recurrence of MDD, treatment resistance, chronicity, or poorer outcome. Although a review of each is beyond the scope of this chapter, their presence suggests the need for extended antidepressant maintenance. Detection of these factors requires early clinical suspicion and specific inquiry.

This matrix-profiling strategy is comparable to that used by cardiologists who consider a cluster of clinical predictors, such as previous risk factors (e.g., smoking, lack of exercise, obesity, previous heart attacks, duration of previous symptoms), family cardiac history, severity of laboratory measures (e.g., blood pressure, cholesterol, isoenzymes, electrocardiography and angiography results), severity of current symptoms (angina, chest pain), and history of previous interventions (e.g., coronary artery bypass graft, stent insertions), when trying to identify patients who require no treatment, maintenance medication, or invasive cardiac intervention.

Once clinical predictors are identified, the next phase is to use the most powerful predictors as independent variables singly and in combination to answer key questions: Which predictors are most powerful? Which combinations have best predictive performance? Which patients are likely to have another episode unless they take medication? Are there any patients who are not at risk even when they are not taking medication? Does risk change over time, and can extended antidepressant medication ever be stopped? If so, when? Can medication doses be lowered without increasing recurrence risk? Are there any long-term dangers of extended antidepressant maintenance medication? Are there differences in effectiveness in recurrence prevention between one type of antidepressant and another? Do gonadal hormone transitions require changes in maintenance treatment strategies? What is the role of augmenting agents in extended maintenance treatment? Are there benefits or risks associated with "maintenance treatment holidays"? Do nutraceuticals such as St.-John's-wort have any role in preventing or precipitating recurrences? How cost-effective are maintenance antidepressant programs? How does poor treatment adherence affect the risk of recurrence?

This list of questions is extensive. There are more. Some are being investigated. Some are discussed in other chapters in the volume, but we still have much to do. As is the case with cardiology, we can reasonably expect the matrix to be refined progressively over the years while clinicians are employing it. However, for such refinement to occur, we must start using it.

Treatment of Recurrent MDD: The Need for Paradigm Shifts

Recommendations for treating patients with recurrent MDD follow (Figure 6–1).

Provide Illness-Focused Treatment

Much as in the treatment of bipolar disorder (see Chapter 4 in this volume), when treating patients with MDD, maintenance treatment should be illness-focused, not episode-focused. An illness focus changes the perspectives of the clinician, patient, and family. It makes everyone think long term. It involves everyone in the monitoring of early warning signs, such as changes in sleep, mood, confidence, appetite, sexual interest, and irritability. It involves everyone in promoting treatment adherence, maintaining structure, and sustaining wellness. And it encourages everyone to become as educated as possible about the disease. This is currently not the focus of care for patients with MDD, even though it is the hallmark of care for patients with bipolar illness. This change will require a large paradigm shift on the part of most clinicians as well as the public.

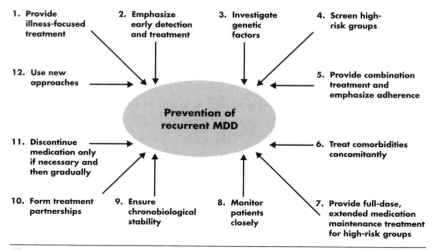

1. Provide illness-focused treatment

2. Emphasize early detection and treatment

3. Investigate genetic factors

4. Screen high-risk groups

12. Use new approaches

5. Provide combination treatment and emphasize adherence

Prevention of recurrent MDD

11. Discontinue medication only if necessary and then gradually

6. Treat comorbidities concomitantly

10. Form treatment partnerships

9. Ensure chronobiological stability

8. Monitor patients closely

7. Provide full-dose, extended medication maintenance treatment for high-risk groups

Figure 6–1. Recommendations for treating patients with recurrent major depressive disorder (MDD)

Emphasize Early Detection and Treatment

Early onset of mood symptoms is not a good sign (Pine et al. 1998). It is often the first ostensible step in a lifelong course of MDD, a pattern of growing disability. Primary care clinicians who note symptoms characteristic of mood disorders in children and adolescents, even if such symptoms are mild and fail to meet severity and duration criteria for the diagnosis of DSM-IV-TR MDD (American Psychiatric Association 2000), should consider that these symptoms may represent the prodromal phase of MDD. As Pine suggested, clinicians and families need to think "mood disorder," not "moodiness." Other diagnoses should not be routinely assigned first, especially if there is a strong family history of depression. Assigning other diagnoses (e.g., "adjustment disorder of adolescence," attention-deficit/hyperactivity disorder) is generally the result of stigma, which delays the onset of effective treatment and launches the growing cascade of burden.

Investigate Genetic Factors

Clinical depression, similar to conditions such as cardiovascular disease and diabetes, has well-documented complex genetic underpinnings (Kendler et al. 1993a, 1993b). These genetic variables are best understood as creating an inherited vulnerability, making it more likely that when susceptible individuals encounter major stressors or life traumas, these variables precipitate underlying neurobiologic abnormalities and an episode of depression (Kendler et al. 1999). Also, as with many other medical conditions, clinical depression involves multiple genes. Such disorders are referred to as complex genetic disorders (Burmeister 1999). The genes interact with environmental events and lifestyle patterns, both of which are important in producing MDD clinical features and a pattern of MDD recurrences.

Comorbidities (e.g., panic disorder, obsessive-compulsive disorder, bulimia) are genetically linked with MDD (Kendler et al. 1993a; Kessler et al. 1994a) and not surprisingly, often respond to the same treatments, such as selective serotonin reuptake inhibitors (SSRIs). Family histories are needed to thoroughly investigate comorbidities as well as dysthymia and MDD.

Screen High-Risk Groups

Because of the higher prevalence of MDD among women, screening must become a priority beginning in adolescence, and should extend into primary care and into children's and women's health care settings. Kendler et al. (1999) assessed the occurrence of 15 classes of major stressors and the onset of MDD during a 1-year period in female twins (24,648 person-months and 316 onsets of MDD) and found that stressful events had a substantial causal relationship with the onset of episodes. The authors concluded that about one-third of the association was noncausal, because the women who were predisposed to MDD selected themselves into high-risk environments, illustrating characteristic stress-genetic interactions. Kessler et al. (1993) pointed out that the higher prevalence of 12-month depression among women is largely the result of women having a higher risk of first onset. Once the sequence has started, the risk for recurrence appears to be greater during transitional times, such as during the postpartum period (see Chapter 2 in this volume).

In geriatric settings, Reynolds et al. (1996a, 1996b) noted that a greater proportion of elderly patients (15.5%) than patients in midlife (6.7%) experienced a relapse during continuation therapy

(P = 0.02) and that relapses occurred earlier in elderly patients (7.4 weeks vs. 16.6 weeks, respectively; P = 0.008). Episodes of relapse in elderly patients also are more confounded with other medical illnesses. Thus, at the opposite end of the age spectrum, when treating elderly patients, more scrutiny is warranted.

Provide Combination Treatment and Emphasize Adherence

"Better, but not well, is not good enough" is a concept that deserves emphasis by clinicians who treat patients with MDD and seek to maintain the patient's wellness (Keller et al. 2000). Treatment resistance is more likely to develop when the patient's condition does not improve; therefore, all necessary measures should be employed to achieve remission, not just symptom improvement, including conducting longer trials with higher doses (a first choice), using augmentation agents, switching across antidepressant classes, switching within the same class, and combining antidepressants.

The clinician should emphasize initial treatment with adequate doses for adequate duration in order to achieve remission and functional improvement, not simply symptom improvement. Adequate duration of treatment warrants special emphasis. As Nierenberg et al. (2000) found, the cumulative probabilities of response at weeks 2, 4, and 6 were 55.5%, 80.2%, and 89.5%, respectively, and patients require at least 4–6 weeks of trial at adequate doses before clinicians can conclude that the treatment is not working.

A large multicenter National Institute of Mental Health study (STAR*D) is under way to test various treatment algorithms for treatment-resistant depression (http://www.edc.gsph.pitt.edu/stard). Valuable information will be generated about which treatment sequences are most likely to work optimally. Meanwhile, as described in Chapter 3 in this volume, even chronically depressed patients showed remarkable progress when vigorously treated with a combination of antidepressant medications and cognitive-behavioral therapy.

Special efforts to enhance treatment adherence (Katon et al. 1999) should be employed whenever possible to sustain remission. Assessment of adherence should be a routine part of treatment for patients whose condition has improved but who remain mildly or moderately symptomatic. To improve adherence, clinicians need to work with patients and families to attack all barriers to long-term use of medications. These include reducing undesirable side effects, the inconvenience of multiple dosing, high costs, and stigma. Medications that can be taken once a day are preferable. Medications that could be taken even less frequently, such as weekly or monthly, might further improve adherence and long-term outcome. Pharmaceutical companies should be encouraged to develop such antidepressants, and clinicians should be encouraged to start initial treatment with those that have been demonstrated to encourage maximal adherence over the long term, thus avoiding unnecessary switches in medication.

As a commentary, the term "adherence" is preferable to "compliance," denoting a partnership rather than an authoritative relationship.

Medication dosage does influence adherence. As noted in Chapter 4 in this volume, adherence is a major concern when treating patients with bipolar disorder and, with a wider range of available treatments, a clinician should test lower doses of any mood stabilizing medication if a patient has experienced even subjective distress as a result of medication. The same advice about lowering dosage *cannot* be given when prescribing extended antidepressant maintenance for patients with MDD, because available data suggest that lowering dosage may increase the risk of recurrence (Kupfer et al. 1992). At some point, clinicians may determine that lower-dose combinations of medications or augmenting agents are as effective as full-dose antidepressant medications, after which lower doses may be possible to minimize side effects. Until then, clinicians are advised to sustain the dose that got the patient better—a full dose.

Treat Comorbidities Concomitantly

As stated previously, MDD is inherently a multifactorial comorbid condition (Kendler et al. 1993a; Kessler et al. 1994a). In addition to depressive symptoms, patients may experience generalized anxiety disorder, panic disorder, phobias, obsessive-compulsive disorder, eating disorders, sleep apnea, psychotic symptoms, and various DSM-IV-TR Axis II disorders, and may abuse alcohol or other substances. It is unknown how such comorbidities influence the course or risk of recurrences, but they greatly accentuate the disabilities associated with MDD. In the past, some believed that one disorder was primary and the other was secondary and that the primary disorder warranted the treatment focus. This led to poorer outcome, lack of adherence, treatment resistance, and growing morbidity. Because some comorbidities, such as adolescent alcohol abuse (De Bellis et al. 2000), also appear to be factors in hippocampal neuronal degeneration, their comorbid presence becomes even more ominous and further emphasizes that *all* comorbid diagnoses should be addressed concomitantly with treatment of MDD. Regardless of how many conditions are present, however, when indicators for indefinite maintenance treatment for recurrent MDD are present (see Table 6–4), maintenance treatment is recommended.

Provide Full-Dose, Extended Medication Maintenance Treatment for High-Risk Groups

A major challenge in implementing full-dose medication maintenance treatment for extended periods is to identify patients at high risk for recurrence. Kraemer et al. (1997) noted that terms such as *risk* and *risk factor* are inconsistently and imprecisely used, and this is also true for the term *risk of recurrence.* Lacking laboratory tests and precise criteria to quantify risk, this task must be clinically driven. In this treatment approach, empirical documentation and clinical evidence provide the foundation for treatment recommendations. These recommendations are derived from the variables listed in Table 6–4 and empirically combined. These variables are combined because they have multiple reports associating them with recurrences, but no studies have precisely quantified their risk potential; no variable appears to handle all circumstances; and few studies have assessed the variables' interactive predictive performance. That research is begging to be completed.

Table 6–4. Guidelines for identifying patients who need indefinite antidepressant treatment for recurrent major depressive disorder (MDD)

Three or more previous episodes of MDD
Two or more previous episodes of MDD, plus one of the following:
    Family history of MDD with at least one family member affected
    More than 120 days spent depressed during lifetime
One or two previous severe episodes of MDD, plus two or more of the following:
    Early age at onset
    Family history of MDD with at least one family member affected
    More than 120 days spent depressed during lifetime
    Treatment resistance
    Psychosis
    Prompt relapse or recurrence following previous discontinuation of treatment
    Previous suicide attempt or persistent suicidal ideation during depressive episodes
    Current severity of episode (e.g., Hamilton Depression Rating Scale score greater than 24)
    Concurrent medical illnesses or personal or occupational circumstances that make any future depressive recurrence truly "hazardous"
    Presence of one or more of the following selected laboratory variables:
        Persistent abnormalities of stress hormone regulation with elevated glucocorticoids or abnormal hypothalamic-pituitary-adrenal measures
        MRI brain imaging evidence of hippocampal or amygdala atrophy not attributable to other causes
        Abnormal electroencephalogram (EEG) sleep assessment, especially low delta sleep ratio (Spanier et al. 1996), diminished slow wave sleep or reduced rapid eye movement (REM) latency (Thase et al. 1994b)

Meanwhile, as a starting point, Table 6–4 lists guidelines for determining which patients should be treated indefinitely with antidepressant medication. As investigators work vigorously to transform these many variables into a matrix of predictors with higher predictive performance (Greden 2000), they still can be used by clinicians to help determine patients at high risk for recurrences. Standardized assessments and routine long-term follow-up are encouraged as high-risk predictors are clinically applied so that we can simultaneously catalyze growth of the database.

Clinical "art" must be used in making MDD treatment decisions, but this is true in making treatment decisions for most major diseases, including diabetes, heart disease, and cancer. From a research perspective, it is important that we begin to test and refine these predictors. From a clinical and public health perspective, it is important that we begin using them.

Once a patient feels better, full doses need to be sustained. As Kupfer (1993) demonstrated, dose reductions lead to recurrences, even after years of successful maintenance treatment. Few studies have assessed whether augmenting strategies prevent relapses, and no studies on this issue have been conducted for any prolonged periods. Bauer et al. (2000), however, studied patients with treatment-refractory MDD and found that none of the 14 patients (0%) who received lithium augmentation with antidepressants experienced a relapse during a double-blind phase of a study, whereas 7 of 15 patients (47%) treated with placebo and antidepressants experienced a relapse. If augmenting agents are required to improve clinical status during acute treatment, their use should be continued during maintenance treatment. If primary care clinicians are uncertain about how to use augmenting agents, they should consider referring patients to specialists before chronicity becomes the status quo.

Because short-term cost considerations for medications have driven treatment decisions, there is pressure to discontinue maintenance treatment after a period of wellness. Yet, when total health care costs and costs to society are considered, such a recommendation appears unwarranted. Kamlet et al. (1993) concluded that "drug maintenance treatment is cost-effective in the strongest sense of the term compared to either a placebo group or interpersonal therapy; it both improves expected lifetime health (measured in quality-adjusted life years, or QALYs) and reduces direct medical costs" (p. 17).

Monitor Patients Closely

Close monitoring of clinical status for any recurrent disorder—even when the patient feels well—is crucial. It is a key part of illness-focused rather than episode-focused care. Patients and families should be involved in selecting forms of monitoring, instructed on how and when to use monitoring scales (e.g., at least weekly), and encouraged to sustain monitoring. Monitoring of symptoms promotes learning and involvement in and ownership of treatment decisions.

When rating scales are being selected, age and educational considerations should play a role. Some patients prefer traditional printed scales, some prefer electronic scales using the Internet or personal digital assistants, and some prefer telephone scales at scheduled intervals with interactive voice recognition. Some patients develop their own scales, and although standardized scales are preferred, these are acceptable as long as they are used consistently. Clinicians should instruct patients and families to make contact when major shifts in symptom severity occur. When a recurrence seems evident, the clinician, patient, and family should be ready to intervene aggressively. In fact, the possibility of this should be discussed beforehand.

Ensure Chronobiological Stability

Chronobiological shifts (e.g., transmeridian travel, major disruptions in sleep, shift work, seasonal transitions) are often precipitants of new MDD episodes. Steps to ensure chronobiological stability must be incorporated into preventive treatment programs. All patients with MDD, especially those who have experienced recurrences, as with patients with bipolar disorder, must be cautioned about the following:

- Careers that require shift work (e.g., police work, nursing, medicine)

- Activities that are erratic (e.g., staying up late to study, attend parties, or use the Internet)
- Transmeridian travel across three or more time zones
- Natural physiological transitions that interfere with sleep (e.g., pregnancy, the postpartum period, menopause)
- Seasonal transitions, especially into winter

Recognizing that many of these are unavoidable, clinicians should recommend active steps to reduce other stressors at vulnerable times, increase the frequency of clinical monitoring and/or concomitant psychotherapy, increase the dosage of antidepressants, and/or start augmenting phototherapy.

Form Treatment Partnerships

The traditional notion of psychiatric consultation needs rethinking when treating patients with MDD. Comanagement of care, in which primary care clinicians work in partnership with psychiatrists and clinicians of other specialties, often in their settings, is recommended (Katon et al. 1999).

In the past, many psychiatrists and other mental health clinicians did not involve family or close partners in treatment decisions because of concerns about patient confidentiality and autonomy. In addition, these clinicians sometimes did not provide family or close partners with requested information. This approach needs to change for treatment of recurrent MDD. Why? A key facet for recurrence prevention is the provision of adequate structure for monitoring and treatment adherence. Family and friends are vital in this. They serve as observers and supporters, provide feedback to clinicians about early recurrence of symptoms, and reiterate the importance of keeping appointments and taking medications to the patient. They also provide valuable input to the patient during discussions about future treatment decisions, often counteracting the patient's negative views of self, world, or future. In effect, families and friends represent a form of ongoing cognitive-behavioral therapy. Mental health clinicians are advised to emulate the treatments used by clinicians treating cancer, diabetes, and heart disease, in which families and others are routinely involved in discussions with the patient. Allies should be recruited, not discouraged. Requests for information should be applauded, not resisted. The more that patients and families know, the better. They are powerful partners in achieving and sustaining wellness. For some clinicians, a paradigm shift will be required for this to occur.

Numerous mental health patient advocacy and support groups have been founded in the United States and elsewhere. These organizations play key roles in public policy legislation and education. Data collected by the National Depressive and Manic-Depressive Association (National DMDA) reveal that patient and family participation also play an important role in encouraging patients to adhere to treatment and in helping families support adherence (Rush 1999). Clinicians should strongly recommend membership in groups such as National DMDA (www.ndmda.org) and the National Alliance for the Mentally Ill (www.nami.org).

Discontinue Medication Only if Necessary and Then Gradually

The risk of recurrences is significantly higher when antidepressants are discontinued (see Table 6–2). The risk appears to intensify when medications are withdrawn suddenly and antidepressant withdrawal syndrome occurs more frequently (Dilsaver 1994; Maixner and Greden 1998). If antidepressant discontinuation cannot be avoided in patients with recurrent depression—and this is an important "if"—a taper of weeks or even months should be planned when possible.

Use New Approaches

Some patients may have MDD recurrences despite best clinical efforts to prevent them. At that point, other approaches should be considered. There is no room for concession to recurrences. The goal remains maintenance of wellness.

Clinicians might first think of using maintenance anticonvulsants (e.g., valproate, lamotrigine, gabapentin) even for patients considered to have unipolar illness, based on the strong possibility that the recurrences are actually cycling episodes in a patient with undiagnosed bipolar II disorder. This occurs commonly. As they appear, other new treatment advances should also be considered.

New approaches are always being explored. For example, Smeraldi et al. (1998) reported that a combination of sleep deprivation, pindolol, and lithium resulted in sustained antidepressant effect in patients with bipolar disorder. The rationale for this treatment is that 1) total sleep deprivation (repeated over three cycles on days 1, 3, and 5) enhances serotonin (5-HT) neurotransmission and reduces sensitivity of the 5-HT_{1A} autoreceptors, 2) pindolol potentiates this action because it is a 5-HT_{1A} blocker, and 3) lithium then presumably maintains the dramatic improvements, perhaps through its own alterations of serotonergic function. Such a strategy has not been studied in patients with unipolar illness but should be.

Maintenance ECT is being employed in many clinical settings. New modalities such as vagus nerve stimulation or repeated transcranial magnetic stimulation (rTMS) might be used singly or in combination with maintenance antidepressants in the future (see Chapter 5 in this volume).

Finally, as we begin genotyping various polymorphisms such as the functional polymorphisms identified for the serotonin transporter (5-HTT) on chromosome 17 (Collier et al. 1996; Mann et al. 2000; Smeraldi et al. 1998), we may determine that different polymorphisms (e.g., l/l, l/s, s/s) require different maintenance antidepressants. Other transporters should also be assessed. Such "culture-and-sensitivity" strategies for selecting the optimal medication have a long tradition in medicine.

Conclusion

MDD is truly burdensome, plaguing millions, diminishing productivity, ruining families, taking lives. But MDD is generally treatable. We are accumulating new knowledge every day, enhancing visibility of the disorder and gradually counteracting the stigma associated with it. We have strong allies, such as the World Health Organization and the U.S. Surgeon General. New knowledge, new treatments, decreased stigma, and strong allies are powerful weapons. Yet we have not made the progress we anticipated.

A prime reason—arguably the key reason—is that MDD is a recurrent disorder. Our clinical target needs to become prevention of new episodes, not just treatment of the current one. We need to protect wellness. We have an array of effective maintenance treatments to accomplish these goals, and we need to begin using them. Prevention of recurrences requires a paradigm shift, a call to arms. The time has come.

References

American Psychiatric Association: Diagnostic and Statistical Manual of Mental Disorders, 4th Edition, Text Revision. Washington, DC, American Psychiatric Association, 2000

Angst J, Baastrup P, Grof P, et al: The course of monopolar depression and bipolar psychoses. Psychiatria, Neurolgia, Neurochirurgia 76: 489–500, 1973

Bauer M, Bschor T, Kunz D, et al: Double-blind, placebo-controlled trial of the use of lithium to augment antidepressant medication in continuation treatment of unipolar major depression. Am J Psychiatry 157:1429–1435, 2000

Bjork K: The efficacy of zimelidine in preventing depressive episodes in recurrent major depressive disorders—a double-blind placebo-controlled study. Acta Psychiatr Scand Suppl 308:182–189, 1983

Burmeister M: Basic concepts in the study of diseases with complex genetics. Biol Psychiatry 45:797–805, 1999

Buysse D, Reynolds C, Hoch C, et al: Longitudinal effects of nortriptyline on EEG sleep and the likelihood of recurrence in elderly depressed patients. Neuropsychopharmacology 14:243–252, 1996

Collier DA, Stober G, Li T, et al: A novel functional polymorphism within the promoter of the serotonin transporter gene: possible role in susceptibility to affective disorders. Mol Psychiatry 1:453–460, 1996

Coppen A, Peet M, Bailey J, et al: Double-blind and open prospective studies on lithium prophylaxis in affective disorders. Psychiatria, Neurolgia, Neurochirurgia 76:500–510, 1973

De Bellis MD, Clark DB, Beers SR, et al: Hippocampal volume in adolescent-onset alcohol use disorders. Am J Psychiatry 157:737–744, 2000

Dilsaver SC: Withdrawal phenomena associated with antidepressant and antipsychotic agents. Drug Saf 10:103–114, 1994

Doogan DP, Caillard V: Sertaline in the prevention of depression. Br J Psychiatry 169:217–222,1992

Frank E, Kupfer DJ: Peeking through the door to the 21st century. Arch Gen Psychiatry 57:83–85, 2000

Frank E, Kupfer DJ, Perel JM, et al: Three-year outcomes for maintenance therapies in recurrent depression. Arch Gen Psychiatry 47: 1093–1099, 1990

Frasure-Smith N, Lesperance F: Coronary artery disease, depression and social support only the beginning. Eur Heart J 21:1043–1045, 2000

Frasure-Smith N, Lesperance F, Gravel G, et al: Social support, depression, and mortality during the first year after myocardial infarction. Circulation 101:1919–1924, 2000

Georgotas A, McCue RE, Cooper TB: A placebo-controlled comparison of nortriptyline and phenelzine in maintenance therapy of elderly depressed patients. Arch Gen Psychiatry 46:783–786, 1989

Glen AIM, Johnson AL, Shepherd M: Continuation therapy with lithium and amitriptyline in unipolar depressive illness: a randomized double-blind controlled trial. Psychol Med 14:37–50, 1984

Goff DC Jr, Feldman HA, McGovern PG, et al: Prehospital delay in patients hospitalized with heart attack symptoms in the United States: the REACT trial. Rapid Early Action for Coronary Treatment (REACT) Study Group. Am Heart J 138:1046–1057, 1999

Goodwin FK, Jamison KR: Course and outcome, in Manic-Depressive Illness. New York, NY, Oxford University Press, 1990, pp 127–156

Greden JF: Antidepressant maintenance medications: when to discontinue and how to stop. J Clin Psychiatry 54:39–45, 1993

Greden JF: Antidepressant maintenance medications, in Pharmacotherapy for Mood, Anxiety, and Cognitive Disorders. Edited by Halbreich U, Montgomery S. Washington, DC, American Psychiatric Press, 2000, pp 315–330

Greden JF, Gardner R, King D, et al: Dexamethasone suppression tests in antidepressant treatment of melancholia. The process of normalization and test-retest reproducibility. Arch Gen Psychiatry 40:493–500, 1983

Ho BC, Andreasen NC, Flaum M, et al: Untreated initial psychosis: its relation to quality of life and symptom remission in first-episode schizophrenia. Am J Psychiatry 157:808–815, 2000

Jakovljevic M, Mewett S: Comparison between paroxetine, imipramine and placebo in preventing recurrent major depressive episodes. Eur Neuropsychopharmacol 1:440, 1991

Kane JM, Quitkin FM, Rifkin A, et al: Lithium carbonate and imipramine in the prophylaxis of unipolar and bipolar II illness: a prospective placebo-controlled comparison. Arch Gen Psychiatry 39: 1065–1069, 1982

Kamlet MS, Paul N, Greenhouse J, et al: Cost utility analysis of maintenance treatment for recurrent depression. Control Clin Trials 16:17–40, 1995

Katon W, Von Korff M, Lin E, et al: Stepped collaborative care for primary care patients with persistent symptoms of depression: a randomized trial. Arch Gen Psychiatry 56:1109–1115, 1999

Keller MB: The long-term treatment of depression. J Clin Psychiatry 60 (suppl 17):41–45; discussion, 46–48, 1999

Keller MB, McCullough JP, Klein DN, et al: A comparison of nefazodone, the cognitive behavioral-analysis system of psychotherapy, and their combination for the treatment of chronic depression. N Engl J Med 342:1462–1470, 2000

Kendler KS, Kessler RC, Neale MC, et al: The prediction of major depression in women: toward an integrated etiologic model. Am J Psychiatry 150:1139–1148, 1993a

Kendler KS, Neale MC, Kessler RC, et al: A longitudinal twin study of 1-year prevalence of major depression in women. Arch Gen Psychiatry 50:843–852, 1993b

Kendler KS, Karkowski LM, Prescott CA: Causal relationship between stressful life events and the onset of major depression. Am J Psychiatry 156:837–841, 1999

Kessler RC, McGonagle KA, Swartz M, et al: Sex and depression in the National Comorbidity Survey. I: lifetime prevalence, chronicity and recurrence. J Affect Disord 29:85–96, 1993

Kessler RC, McGonagle KA, Nelson CB, et al: Sex and depression in the National Comorbidity Survey. II: cohort effects. J Affect Disord 30:15–26, 1994a

Kessler RC, McGonagle KA, Zhao S, et al: Lifetime and 12-month prevalence of DSM-III-R psychiatric disorders in the United States: results from the National Comorbidity Survey. Arch Gen Psychiatry 51:8–19, 1994b

Kraemer HC, Kazdin A, Offord D, et al: Coming to terms with the terms of risk. Arch Gen Psychiatry 54:337–343, 1997

Kupfer DJ: Maintenance treatment in recurrent depression: current and future directions. The first William Sargant Lecture. Br J Psychiatry 161:309–316, 1992

Kupfer DJ: Management of recurrent depression. J Clin Psychiatry 54 (2, suppl):29–33, 1993

Kupfer DJ, Frank E, Perel JM, et al: Five-year outcome for maintenance therapies in recurrent depression. Arch Gen Psychiatry 49:769–773, 1992

Kupfer DJ, Ehlers CL, Frank E, et al: Persistent effects of antidepressants: EEG sleep studies in depressed patients during maintenance treatment. Biol Psychiatry 35:781–793, 1994

Lieberman JA: Is schizophrenia a neurodegenerative disorder? A clinical and neurobiological perspective. Biol Psychiatry 46:729–739, 1999

Lieberman JA, Fenton WS: Delayed detection of psychosis: causes, consequences, and effect on public health. Am J Psychiatry 157:1727–1730, 2000

Maixner SM, Greden JF: Extended antidepressant maintenance and discontinuation syndromes. Depress Anxiety 8 (suppl 1):43–53, 1998

Mann JJ, Huang YY, Underwood MD, et al: A serotonin transporter gene promoter polymorphism (5-HTTLPR) and prefrontal cortical binding in major depression and suicide. Arch Gen Psychiatry 57:729–738, 2000

McGlashan TH: Duration of untreated psychosis in first episode schizophrenia: marker or determinant of course. Biol Psychiatry 46:899–907, 1999

Montgomery SA, Dunbar GC: Paroxetine is better than placebo in relapse prevention and the prophylaxis of recurrent depression. Int Clin Psychopharmacol 8:189–195, 1993

Montgomery SA, Dufour H, Brion S, et al: The prophylactic efficacy of fluoxetine in unipolar depression. Br J Psychiatry 153 (suppl 3):69–76, 1988

Murray CJL, Lopez AD: The Global Burden of Disease: A Comprehensive Assessment of Mortality and Disability From Disease, Injuries, and Risk Factors in 1990 and Projected to 2020, Vol 1. Cambridge, MA, World Health Organization/Harvard University Press, 1996

Nierenberg AA, Amsterdam JD: Treatment-resistant depression: definition and treatment approaches. J Clin Psychiatry 51 (6, suppl):39–47, 1990

Nierenberg AA, Farabaugh AH, Alpert JE, et al: Timing of onset of antidepressant response with fluoxetine treatment. Am J Psychiatry 157:1423–1428, 2000

Perlis M, Giles D, Buysse D, et al: Self-reported sleep disturbance as a prodromal symptom in recurrent depression. J Affect Disord 42:209–212, 1997

Pfeffer C: The Suicidal Child. New York, Guilford, 1986

Pine DS, Cohen P, Gurley D, et al: The risk for early adulthood anxiety and depressive disorders in adolescents with anxiety and depressive disorders. Arch Gen Psychiatry 55:56–64, 1998

Prien RF, Klett J, Caffey EM Jr: Lithium carbonate and imipramine in prevention of affective episodes: report from the NIMH collaborative study of lithium therapy. Arch Gen Psychiatry 29:420–425, 1973

Prien RF, Kupfer DJ, Mansky PA, et al: Drug therapy in the prevention of recurrences in unipolar and bipolar affective disorders. Report of the NIMH Collaborative Study Group comparing lithium carbonate, imipramine, and a lithium carbonate–imipramine combination. Arch Gen Psychiatry 41:1096–1104, 1984

Reynolds CF III, Frank E, Kupfer DJ, et al: Treatment outcome in recurrent major depression: a post hoc comparison of elderly ("young old") and midlife patients. Am J Psychiatry 153:1288–1292, 1996a

Reynolds CF III, Frank E, Perel JM, et al: High relapse rate after discontinuation of adjunctive medication for elderly patients with recurrent major depression. Am J Psychiatry 153:1418–1422, 1996b

Roan: Redefining what we call a "heart attack." Los Angeles Times, September 18, 2000

Robinson DS, Lerfald SC, Bennett B, et al: Continuation and maintenance treatment of major depression with the monoamine oxidase inhibitor phenelzine: a double-blind placebo-controlled discussion study. Psychopharmacol Bull 27:31–39, 1991

Rouillon F, Serrurier D, Miller H, et al: Prophylactic efficacy of maprotiline on unipolar depression relapse. J Clin Psychiatry 52:423–431, 1991

Rush JT: National DMDA Support Group Survey: Does Participation in a Support Group Increase Treatment Compliance? Chicago, IL, National Depressive and Manic-Depressive Association, 1999

Schou M: Lithium Research at the Psychopharmacology Research Unit, Risskov, Denmark: A Historical Account in Origin, Prevention and Treatment of Affective Disorders. Edited by Schou M, Stromgren E. London, Academic Press, 1979, pp 1–8

Sheline Y, Wang P, Gado M, et al: Hippocampal atrophy in recurrent major depression. Proc Natl Acad Sci U S A 93:3908–3913, 1996

Sheline YI, Gado MH, Price JL: Amygdala core nuclei volumes are decreased in recurrent major depression. Neuroreport 9:2023–2028, 1998

Sheline YI, Sanghavi M, Mintun MA, et al: Depression duration but not age predicts hippocampal volume loss in medically healthy women with recurrent major depression. J Neurosci 19:5034–5043, 1999

Smeraldi E, Zanardi R, Benedetti F, et al: Polymorphism within the promoter of the serotonin transporter gene and antidepressant efficacy of fluvoxamine. Mol Psychiatry 3:508–511, 1998

Spanier C, Frank E, McEachran AB, et al: The prophylaxis of depressive episodes in recurrent depression following discontinuation of drug therapy: integrating psychological and biological factors. Psychol Med 26:461–475, 1996

Starkman MN, Giordani B, Gebarski SS, et al: Decrease in cortisol reverses human hippocampal atrophy following treatment of Cushing's disease. Biol Psychiatry. 46:1595–1602, 1999

Thase ME, Reynolds CF III, Frank E, et al: Do depressed men and women respond similarly to cognitive behavior therapy? Am J Psychiatry 151:500–505, 1994a

Thase ME, Reynolds CF III, Frank E, et al: Polysomnographic studies of unmedicated depressed men before and after cognitive behavioral therapy. Am J Psychiatry 151:1615–1622, 1994b

Wyatt RJ: Neuroleptics and the natural course of schizophrenia. Schizophr Bull 17:325–351, 1991

Zis AP, Goodwin FK: Major affective disorder as a recurrent illness: a critical review. Arch Gen Psychiatry 36 (8, Spec No):835–839, 1979a

Zis AP, Goodwin FK: Novel antidepressants and the biogenic amine hypothesis of depression. The case for iprindole and mianserin. Arch Gen Psychiatry 36:1097–1107, 1979b

Index

Page numbers printed in **boldface** *type refer to tables or figures.*

Geriatric Depression Study,
71–72, 75
Gonadal hormones
and adolescent-onset
depression, 21
perimenopausal levels of, and
mood, 44–45

Headache, in adolescent
depression, 22, 23
Health care costs, of depression,
1–2
Heart disease, and major
depressive disorder,
comparison of, 143–146, **145**
Herbal remedies, use in
pregnancy, 34–35
High-risk groups, for recurrent
depression, 14–15
identification of, 158, **159,** 160
maintenance treatment for,
158–161
screening of, 155–156
Hippocampus, neuronal
degeneration in, in
depression, 13–14
Hormone replacement therapy
(HRT)
antidepressant effect of, in
midlife, 45–47
as augmentation strategy, in
midlife depression, 47
Hypericum perforatum, use in
pregnancy, 34
Hypersomnia, in adolescent
depression, 23
Hypomania. *See* Bipolar disorder
Hypothalamic-pituitary-
adrenocortical axis, effect of
adverse experiences on, 7–8,
21–22

Hypothyroidism, postpartum,
and depression, 27–28

Imipramine
for chronic depression,
outcome with, 64–65, **66**
in combination therapy, 67–69,
69–71, **70**
and lithium, combined,
maintenance treatment
with, outcome of, 62, **64**
maintenance treatment with,
outcome of, 62, **64**
in prevention of recurrent
depression, versus
placebo, **148**
Infanticide, postpartum
depression and, 39
Inositol, 97
Insomnia, in adolescent
depression, 23
Interpersonal psychotherapy,
and pharmacotherapy,
combined
for depression, 69–71, **70**
for recurrent depression in
elderly, 71–72, 75
Irritability, in adolescent
depression, 22

Lactation
antidepressants and, **32–33,**
38–39
FDA categorization of
psychotropic medication
use during, **36–37**
Lamotrigine
adverse effects and side effects
of, 95–96
for bipolar disorder, 95–96
and valproate, combined, 96

Light, increased exposure to, and relapse of bipolar disorder, 84–85
Lithium
adverse effects and side effects of, management of, 85–86
and antidepressant, efficacy of, 160
for bipolar disorder, 90, 92–95
and carbamazepine, comparison of, 92
continuation rates with, 93
depressive symptoms and, 93
maintenance therapy with, 92–95
manic symptoms and, 93
outcomes with, 93
poor response to, predictors of, 93, **94**
response to, medications that improve, 93, **94**
and valproate, comparison of, 90–91, **92**
and carbamazepine combined, 96
comparison of, 96
developmental risks associated with, **32**
discontinuation of, 88, 94
in pregnancy, and recurrent bipolar disorder, 28
dosage and administration of, 86, 94–95
and imipramine, combined, maintenance treatment with, outcome of, 62, **64**
in lactating women, **32**, 38
maintenance treatment with, 85
dosage and administration of, 94–95

outcome of, 62, **64**
neonatal toxicity of, **32**, 35
neuroprotective effects of, 14
and olanzapine, combined, for bipolar disorder, 97
with pindolol and sleep deprivation, in treatment of bipolar disorder, 164
in prevention of recurrent depression, versus placebo, **148–149**
response to, factors affecting, 85
and risperidone, combined, for bipolar disorder, 97
teratogenicity of, **32,** 35
use in pregnancy, 35, 38

Magnetic resonance imaging (MRI), of brain, in mood disorders, 13–14
Magnetic seizure therapy, 108–109
clinical applicability of, **107,** 109
invasiveness of, **107**
regional specificity of, **107,** 109
Maintenance treatment
for bipolar disorder, 89–90
goals of, 81
keeping patient in, 85–87
for depression. *See also* Pittsburgh Maintenance Therapies in Recurrent Depression
adherence to, 11–12, 90, 156–157
cost-effectiveness of, 160–161
current attitudes toward, 11
dosage and administration of, 158–161

Maintenance treatment
(continued)
for depression *(continued)*
efficacy of, 61–65, **63**
for high-risk groups,
158–161
historical perspective on,
10–11
illness-focused, 153
new approaches to, 163–164
outcome of, 61–65, **64**
patients requiring,
identification of, 158,
159, 160
in prevention of recurrent
depression, 147
research on, need for,
146–147
Major depressive disorder
(MDD). *See also* Depression
age-related prevalence of, 41,
42
disability caused by, 1
comorbidities and, 158
longitudinal course of, 8–10, **9**
and other chronic disorders,
comparison of, 143–146,
145
personal burden of, 1–2
reduction of, strategies for,
14–15
in pregnancy
case example of, 39–40
clinical features of, 29
fetal effects of, 30
maternal effects of, 29–30
and obstetric outcome, 30
prevalence of, 27–28
research on, need for, 49
risk factors for, 28–29
sequelae of, 29–30

treatment of, 30–35
prevalence of, 3
in adolescents, 4, 20
by age group, 41, **42**
in children, 4
in men, 3
in pregnancy, 27–28
in women, 3, 19
prevention of
in adolescents, 24, 48
in women, research on,
need for, 48–50
recurrence of. *See*
Recurrence(s), of
depression
societal burden of, 1–2, **3**
reduction of, strategies for,
14–15
treatment of. *See* Treatment, of
depression
understanding of, historical
perspective on, 10–11
Mania. *See* Bipolar disorder
Maprotiline, in prevention of
recurrent depression, versus
placebo, **148**
Matrix-profiling strategy, for
identification of at-risk
patients, 150–152
Medical disorders, and relapse of
bipolar disorder, 83–84, **84**
Memory, studies of, vagus nerve
stimulation in, 129–130
Men. *See also* Sex differences
prevalence of depression in, 3
Menopause
age at, 40
definition of, 40
and depression, 40–42
onset of, antidepressant
treatment and, 45

Nonadherence to treatment. *See also* Adherence
in adolescents, 25
Noncompliance with treatment. *See* Adherence
Nortriptyline
in combination therapy, for depression in elderly, 71–72
in prevention of recurrent depression, versus placebo, **149**
Nucleus tractus solitarius (NTS), vagus nerve and, 121–123, **122**

Obesity, treatment of, vagus nerve stimulation in, 129
Obsessive-compulsive disorder (OCD)
as comorbid diagnosis in depression, 158
deep brain stimulation in, 134
transcranial magnetic stimulation in, 117
Obsessive symptoms, and adolescent depression, 23
Olanzapine
for bipolar disorder, 90, 97
dosage and administration of, 97
and lithium, combined, for bipolar disorder, 97
and valproate, combined, for bipolar disorder, 97
Omega-3 fatty acids, 97

Pain, treatment of, vagus nerve stimulation in, 129
Panic disorder, as comorbid diagnosis in depression, 158

Parkinson's disease, deep brain stimulation in, 130–134
Paroxetine
continuation treatment with, outcome of, 62, **63**
in prevention of recurrent depression, versus placebo, **149**
Perimenopause
definition of, 42
and depression, 40–42
estrogen therapy in, antidepressant effect of, 45–47
women at risk for depression in, 44
Pharmacotherapy
for adolescent depression, 25–26
for bipolar disorder, 89–97
combination treatment in, 97–98
for depression. *See also* Antidepressant(s); Psychotherapy, and pharmacotherapy, combined
augmenting agents with, 160
discontinuation of, 163
long-term, 61–65
and onset of menopause, 45
responsivity to, in women, research on, need for, 48
for prevention of recurrent depression, 146–147, **148–149**
tolerability of, importance of, 90
Phenelzine, in prevention of recurrent depression, versus placebo, **148–149**

Psychotherapy. *See also* Cognitive
therapy
for adolescent depression, 24
for bipolar patients, 87–89
brief, as preventive strategy,
need for research on, 49
and pharmacotherapy,
combined, 59, 65–74, 156
benefits of, 75–76
for chronic depression,
72–74, **73**
cost-benefit analysis of,
74–75
for depression in elderly,
71–72, 75
differential effects of, on
specific symptoms, 75
economic analysis of, 76
medication best suited for,
77
for midlife depression, 47
patients best suited for, 77
versus pharmacotherapy
alone, 74
in pregnancy, 38
in prevention of recurrent
depression, 147
providers for, 76
psychotherapeutic approach
best suited for, 77
versus psychotherapy
alone, 74
research on, need for, 77–78
for postpartum depression, 39
in prevention of recurrent
depression, 147
Puerperal psychosis. *See*
Psychosis, postpartum

Race, and depression, 22
Rating scales, 161

Recurrence(s), of bipolar
disorder. *See* Bipolar
disorder, recurrence of
Recurrence(s), of depression
acceleration of, **9,** 10
clinical variables associated
with, 150–152
epidemiological variables
associated with, 150–152
frequent, 8–10, **9**
genetic vulnerability to, 7–8
high-risk groups for, 14–15
identification of, 158, **159,**
160
maintenance treatment for,
158–161
screening of, 155–156
laboratory tests for, 150–152
length of, **9,** 10
midlife depression as, 43–45
patients at risk for,
identification of, 150–152
postpartum, prevalence of, 28
prevalence of, 60
prevention of. *See* Prevention
rates of, 43, 61
research on, need for, 150–153,
151
in women, 48–50
risk factors for, 61, 155
research on, need for, 158
treatment of. *See* Pittsburgh
Maintenance Therapies in
Recurrent Depression;
Treatment
in women, 19–50
Relapse, of depression
in elderly, 155–156
midlife depression as, 43–45
prediction of, brain imaging in,
104

Sertraline
for chronic depression,
outcome with, 64–65, **66**
continuation treatment with,
outcome of, 62, **63**
in lactating women, 39
in prevention of recurrent
depression, versus
placebo, **149**
Sex differences. *See also* Men;
Women
in adolescent depression, 20–22
in age at onset, 43
in cigarette smoking, in
adolescent depression, 23
in genetic vulnerability to
depression, 21
in recurrence rates, 43
in response to SSRIs, 7–8
in stress response, 7
in suicide, in adolescent
depression, 22
Sexual abuse, and depression,
21–22
Signs and symptoms of
depression
in adolescence, 22–23
early detection of, 154
monitoring of, in patients at
risk for recurrence, 161
onset of
early, 4–5, 20
sex differences in, 4–5, 20
timing of, 4, 20
perimenopausal, 41, 42, 44
postpartum, 29
Sleep
disturbances of
in adolescent depression, 23
perimenopausal, and mood,
44

inadequate, and relapse of
bipolar disorder, 83
vagus nerve stimulation and,
129
Sleep apnea, as comorbid
diagnosis in depression,
158
Sleep deprivation
for depression, prediction of
response to, brain imaging
in, 104
with pindolol and lithium, in
treatment of bipolar
disorder, 164
Socioeconomic status, of women
with early-onset depression,
4, 20
Somatic symptoms
in adolescent depression, 22,
23
perimenopausal, and
depression, 41, 42, 44
STAR*D, 156
Stigma, of depression, 11–12
trends in, 25
Stimulants, and bipolar disorder,
83–84
Stomach pain, in adolescent
depression, 23
Stress-genetic interactions, 155
Stressor(s)
and depression in women, 155
and midlife depression in
women, 40, 43
research on, need for, 49
neuronal degeneration caused
by, 13–14
and recurrence of depression,
7–8
and relapse of bipolar
disorder, 85